FORGOTTEN PEOPLE:
POSITIVE APPROACHES TO DEMENTIA CARE

For our families, colleagues and friends

Forgotten People: Positive Approaches to Dementia Care

Jonathan Parker
Bridget Penhale
School of Community and Health Studies,
University of Hull

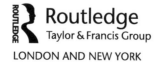

Routledge
Taylor & Francis Group

LONDON AND NEW YORK

First published 1998 by Ashgate Publishing

Reissued 2018 by Routledge
2 Park Square, Milton Park, Abingdon, Oxon, OX14 4RN
711 Third Avenue, New York, NY 10017

Routledge is an imprint of the Taylor & Francis Group, an informa business

Notice:
Product or corporate names may be trademarks or registered trademarks, and are used only for identification and explanation without intent to infringe.

Publisher's Note
The publisher has gone to great lengths to ensure the quality of this reprint but points out that some imperfections in the original copies may be apparent.

Disclaimer
The publisher has made every effort to trace copyright holders and welcomes correspondence from those they have been unable to contact.

A Library of Congress record exists under LC control number: 97049445

Typeset by Manton Typesetters, 5–7 Eastfield Road, Louth, Lincolnshire, LN11 7AJ, UK.

ISBN 13: 978-1-138-31656-0 (hbk)
ISBN 13: 978-1-138-31657-7 (pbk)
ISBN 13: 978-0-429-45557-5 (ebk)

Contents

List of figures

List of boxes

Introduction

There is a surge of interest in dementia care from an academic and practice-focused point of view. There is a growing, almost palpable, anxiety throughout Europe about the millennium and social and economic needs resulting from an ageing population. There are fears for care and support from official bodies and social services, from the family and from private resources. Uncertainties abound, and much is discussed.

Not all is bleak, and there is also a great deal of optimism and excitement about the possibilities for future care practice in the social and health domains. Whilst both the authors are employed as academics, we have also practised social work for people with dementia and their caregivers. We have worked with the pain and the joy such experiences can bring. The aim of this book is to promote social work practice that sees the person first and starts from a clear value base of respect. We have drawn on some of our many experiences and provide illustrations of the positive work that can be done with people to promote a sense of well-being and, as far as possible, partnership.

In this present climate it may be argued that a book which outlines a range of theoretical approaches is outdated and what we need now is a procedural and more bureaucratic approach to social work practice. It might be said that this fits much more comfortably with care management and the newly 'down-sized' social services departments which increasingly adopt a purer commissioning role. If this was all social work was about, we might agree. However, social work is about finding that fit between personal, familial and social need and the demands and responsibilities society places on its citizens. Social workers negotiate a tense tightrope between individual and society. They are concerned with citizenship and the reciprocal flow of responsibilities and rights. In order to achieve this difficult task, practitioners need not only clear and effective procedures but tools and models that can illuminate paths to tread with people through demanding times. The models, approaches and 'tools' we discuss provide just such an array. Like any toolkit, of course, they need to be employed appropriately, used for the right job and in a way that is skilled, safe and constructive. Social workers must operate from a clear value base which emphasises the dignity and personhood of individuals. The way an approach is used needs to be judged against this.

The book is divided into two parts. In Part I the context and background to dementia care is introduced, setting the scene for the presentation of a range of methods and approaches for practice in Part II. The methods are separated into three broad themes: action-focused and behavioural approaches, talking and counselling approaches, and more politically oriented methods. Of course, these often overlap – the separation we impose is for illustrative purposes and in no way implies that validating the worth and humanity of a person with dementia does not constitute a vital part of a task-centred approach to practice, for example.

In writing this book, we seek to champion the rights and responsibilities of people with dementia and the social work practitioners who work alongside them, and to add a small part to the important growing movement towards effective, competent practice that is underpinned by values which respect personhood and promote a person's choices in life. The debate concerning the use of models and approaches in social work rages on. It is clear that some practitioners still do not consciously and judiciously use the tools in their toolkit but rely on an intuitive 'feel' for the situation. Whilst this may be right in some circumstances, it is not underpinned by evidence – and if it is not systematic, it is hardly accountable practice. An explicit use of the models and approaches of value to social work will assist in making practice open to scrutiny and more of a genuine partnership. When working for people with dementia, the need to be accountable is strong. They may not be able to challenge practice for themselves.

The following case study provides an illustration of some of the reasons why we wrote this book.

CASE STUDY: JANET AND MARK

Janet and Mark Palphramand lived on the seventh floor of a large tower block just to the west of the city centre. They had lived there since it was built in 1969, and felt strongly that it was their home. They had been offered alternative accommodation in sheltered housing. It was believed that this would help Janet look after Mark since a recent stroke which had affected his mobility and speech. He also suffered from dementia, and had done so for a number of years.

When visiting, the social worker was asked: 'You're not from social services are you? The last one they sent seemed to sit there and listen but do the opposite to what we'd asked. All we want is help to get over this bad patch. But I want to know you *know* what you're doing.'

There are so many people to thank in connection with the writing of this book. To name them all would be impossible. Perhaps our greatest thanks should go to those people with whom we have worked over the years. They have inspired, saddened and yet heartened us. They are the people who make positive approaches to dementia care possible.

Part I

The context for practice

The first part of this book sets the scene for contemporary social work in dementia care. Social work has gone through many changes in recent years. Some of these have been legislative, such as the implementation of the National Health Service and Community Care Act 1990 and the Carers (Recognition and Services) Act 1995. These changes have influenced policy and procedure in local authority social services departments throughout England and Wales, and similar upheavals have occurred in Scotland. Local government reorganisation has affected the delivery of social services and has consequences for the setting of priorities. All these higher-level changes influence the way social workers practise.

At the level of training, the introduction and revision of the Diploma in Social Work and the corresponding emphasis on competence for practice have again had a tremendous impact on what social workers learn, and consequently what they do in practice. The debate concerning professional education and training continues and is important to the pursuit of good ethical practice. However, in Part I we will introduce changes in the way dementia is approached and understood. Although the medical model remains predominant in the minds of many practitioners, care staff and for the general public, new approaches are gaining ground which encourage optimism regarding the quality of care and well-being that can be achieved for people with dementia and their carers. Chapter 1 will detail both traditional and developing models of dementia to set the stage for understanding. In the next two chapters this will be put into the context of policy and procedural change and developments in training for social work.

1 What is dementia, and why are social workers involved?

Introduction

In the latter decades of the twentieth century there has been a tremendous shift in our understanding of social and health issues, and there have been corresponding developments with respect to dementia and ageing. We no longer automatically associate ageing with dementia, although increasing public knowledge of the condition has led to fears, concerns and beliefs that lead to further problems. Demographic and social changes have raised questions of care, family and individual responsibility which, in their turn, have created political and social debate about systems of welfare. Whilst research indicates clearly that family care and responsibility is as strong as earlier in the century (Parker, 1990; Twigg et al., 1990; Finch, 1989), the context of care and the impact it has upon individuals is well recognised and fuels the welfare debate.

This chapter will provide an overview of the context in which work with people with dementia and their families is carried out. The impact of dementia on those involved will be examined. Following on from this, we shall briefly introduce some of the models proposed for understanding dementia, and suggest that an integrated model proves the most useful for social work practice. Finally, we turn to a brief consideration of the caregiving role and the location of social work practice within the context described. This will form a link to Chapter 2, which deals with the development of community care and care management and the context of dementia.

3

Overview and impact of dementia

Improvements in health and welfare provision throughout the twentieth century, but particularly in the post-war era, have meant that the number of older people surviving into late old age has increased steadily. Life expectancy for men and women has also increased, although women can still expect to live longer than men by an average of some seven years and more women than men survive into old age (Arber and Ginn, 1991). This has been accompanied by an apparent increase in vulnerability: the incidence of disability also increases with age. This is not to say that all older people are frail and vulnerable, or that all older people will suffer from one or more disabilities, but that the likelihood increases with age.

. The incidence of dementia also increases as people become older and live longer (see Marshall, 1996). Whilst the incidence of dementia is around 5 per cent at age 60, 20 per cent of who are aged 80 and over can expect to develop dementia (Jorm, 1987). Whilst this figure and the increased likelihood of developing the illness with age is of concern to many, it needs to be kept in perspective: 80 per cent of those aged 80 or over *do not* develop dementia.

In conjunction with this, figures are available concerning the provision of residential care for older people: this is fairly consistently acknowledged as being at around 5 per cent for those who survive into 'old old age' (over 80 years) (Allen et al., 1992). Therefore, 95 per cent of very elderly people do not live in or enter residential care and do not end their days 'in care'. The majority of older people remain living in the community, mostly in their own homes, being cared for, if necessary, by relatives and members of the family.

Increased geographical mobility and demographic changes (more divorces, more women in the workforce, more lone-parent families) have altered the profile in recent decades somewhat so that more informal networks of care may be less evident than previously. However, the majority of older people neither develop dementia nor require care provided by the state.

Within this overall context, it is also necessary to be aware that social and healthcare practitioners do not work with the majority of individuals, and that we work with individuals and situations that are or have become problematic for one reason or another. It is precisely the fact that we are principally involved with people for whom life has become difficult, if not impossible, that can lead to the development of some regrettable attitudes and notions concerning older people among care professionals. Institutionalised ageism is alive and well in health and social care organisations (Jack, 1992) and needs to be recognised and addressed by all those concerned.

For those individuals who do develop dementia and do require assistance and support from us, we need to remain sensitive to their needs and able to respond to them as individuals. Whether it is the person with dementia, their family or their wider network which is in need of assistance, this should be provided in ways which are consistent with principles of empowerment and anti-oppressive practice. These should maximise opportunities for the person with dementia to be as self-determining and as independent for as long as possible, and decision-making capabilities should always be promoted for the individual concerned.

This can be a delicate and complicated area with caregivers and other family members who may assume natural rights to take decisions on behalf of impaired individuals; it will undoubtedly require skill and great sensitivity on the part of the practitioner in order to handle such situations effectively. Remembering the uniqueness of each individual's circumstances and situation, and working to empower and enable (rather than to protect) are useful and necessary tools in this type of work.

Nevertheless, the potential impact of dementia on individuals and their families should not be underestimated. Dementia is a progressive and terminal illness from which people do not, at present, recover. Its effects are irreversible (although they may be slowed down) and devastating. The impact in terms of workload and costs to health and social care organisations is significant, partly because of the numbers of individuals who are affected (although a relatively small proportion of the total older population, it is still a large number). The impact in terms of the effect on individuals and their families is, in our view, potentially of greater magnitude and includes such possible reactions as anticipatory grief and sorrow at the situation and the perceived loss of the individual as the condition progresses.

It is not possible to understand fully what a person with dementia experiences, although some valuable work in exploring this area has been taking place (Kitwood, 1990; Gilliard, 1997). However, as care practitioners we can listen, empathise and respond to individuals, whether they are the person with dementia or the caregiver. We can also draw on our own personal experiences in this area, where appropriate, although we must remain wary of over-identifying with individuals and their situations, and must remain separate and objective enough to really assist people. It is also crucial to retain a clear sense of who the person we are working with is at any point in time, what we are working to achieve, and what the impact of the illness is on a particular system and network of individuals. What we must also bear in mind is that this is likely to change over time, and we must always remain alert to this probability and to the nature of the potential impacts of dementia in our dealings with individuals.

Understanding dementia: The models

At first glance dementia may seem easy to understand and define, but there are many ways to approach it. The medical model is most widely accepted and understood, and considers dementia in terms of disease and illness or something being wrong in part of the body – in this case the brain. But to ignore other ways of considering the condition, concept or label is dangerous because it does not allow for an approach which acknowledges the uniqueness and worth of the individual, and this is what is important in the delivery of social work and social care.

This section will outline a range of sociological and psychological approaches to dementia that provide alternatives to the accepted models developed within medical settings. We will suggest that no single approach can explain dementia satisfactorily. Rather, an understanding which integrates medical, sociological and psychological thinking is best when seeking to offer help and support to people with dementia and their families. The following topics will be covered:

- *the medical model* – definitions, characteristics, clinical features and diseases causing dementia
- *sociological approaches* – structuralist, interactionist and ethnomethodological approaches
- *a psychosocial model*.

Activity 1.1

Before reading the rest of this section, note down your understanding of dementia. How do you define it? Can you pinpoint where your understanding comes from and how it developed? Keep these notes, as it will be useful to return to them throughout this chapter.

The medical model

Advances in public health medicine, vaccination, antibiotics and drug treatments, and the development of a strong organisational and professional base have ensured that the medical profession has established and maintained a high profile and a great deal of respect in the public mind in the Western world (Turner, 1987). We place our trust in doctors when threatened or incapacitated by disease, and it is a 'cure' we seek or expect when suffering from a condition described, diagnosed and dealt with by them. This model reflects a linear process mediated by a medical practitioner, as shown in Figure 1.1.

Illness → Medical practitioner → Cure

Figure 1.1 The linear process of the medical model

Mental and physical health are often described as branches of the same tree, and approached with similar methods and skills. They are differentiated only by their specific knowledge bases. It is not surprising, therefore, that most people regard dementia as a clearly recognisable and describable medical condition. Whilst there are some problems with accepting this at face value – pathology differs from sufferer to sufferer and clinical presentation is unique to each individual – it is important to understand how the medical profession approaches dementia in general. Social work practitioners operate with a wide range of disciplines and professions. In order to execute their duties successfully it is important to be conversant with the approaches and models employed by others. However, the medical model leads to optimism about 'curing' or at least retarding progress, as seen in Figure 1.2. Although medical advances continue, this view is not borne out in practice, and may create false hopes. At first this may be necessary while people adjust to the implications of the diagnosis, but the search for a cure may detract from the search for quality of care in the longer term.

Dementia → Illness → Medical practitioner → Cure

Figure 1.2 The misplaced hope of the 'pure' medical model

Definitions

The Royal College of Physicians (1981) was concerned that all older people were being characterised by memory impairment, incapacity and loss of control. To counteract these misunderstandings it produced a report describing a variety of syndromes and the causes, or *aetiology*, of organic mental impairment in older people. The following operational definition of dementia resulted:

> Dementia is the global impairment of higher cortical functions including memory, the capacity to solve the problems of day-to-day living, the performance of learned perceptuo-motor skills, the correct use of social skills and control of emotional reactions, in the absence of gross clouding of consciousness. The condition is often irreversible and progressive. (Royal College of Physicians, 1981, p. 146)

This kind of definition is generally accepted in medical circles (Gelder et al., 1989; Lishman, 1987). Dementia represents a deterioration of previously normal functioning as a result of underlying brain damage or disease. The definition is tightly packed and needs some explaining. Firstly, dementia affects all the person's thinking and problem-solving abilities: it is global. The impairment results in a progressive deterioration of all learned skills important for daily living, interacting and communicating with others and functioning as an individual.

This approach firmly places dementia within the province of the medical profession. Correct diagnosis of the disease is essential in deciding possible treatments, especially for reversible conditions and acute confusional states (Wilcock, 1990). It is important in making a prognosis and seeking appropriate medical care. Thus some argue for a precise definition describing a progressive condition associated with detectable neuronal or other structural brain pathology (Levy and Post, 1982). If it is progressive and cannot be halted, however, the hope associated with the medical model cannot be justified. Such a discrete approach is not held by most medical practitioners.

The psychiatrist Elaine Murphy (1986) adds to this debate her observation that an understanding of the uniqueness of each individual sufferer is important. She states that symptoms vary from person to person. This depends on a number of factors, including the site and progress of the disease in the brain and how the individual reacts to and copes with the situation. So the medical model does not preclude a consideration of individuals, their personalities and unique wants and needs. It is important to bear this in mind so that we do not ignore the importance and value of the medical model.

The importance of accurate diagnosis and definition of dementia is seen in *epidemiology*, the study of incidence and prevalence of disease in specified areas, especially in planning public and policy responses to deal with disease.

In 1986 Henderson undertook a wide survey concerning the epidemiology of Alzheimer's disease, to consider risk factors, add to the clinical picture, to provide information for policymakers, and to construct instruments for the study of dementia. Prevalence was difficult to determine because of differences in the age of the study sample, variations in living status, regional differences, lack of differentiation between diagnostic types, and also a lack of standardised diagnostic criteria.

In a review article, Kay (1991) reports a prevalence rate of 1–8 per cent among the population aged 65 years and over. Prevalence rises with age. Incidence studies require assessment at two distinct points in time, and relatively few have been carried out. In the studies that are available, the rate appears to treble for each additional ten years of age over 65 years.

Such studies are rare and difficult to assess, for the same reasons mentioned in relation to prevalence rates. In order for doctors to establish accurate prevalence and incidence figures, and for them to be any use, it is essential that they know what they are looking for.

Activity

Return to your original thoughts concerning dementia. In the light of the definitions provided by the medical model, can you say how these have influenced your understanding? What feelings are aroused by considering dementia as a disease – something being wrong or not working correctly in the person's brain? Does this have any implications for your approach to your work with people suffering from dementia?

Comments

Perhaps you have thought about how you respond when you first learn a person has dementia and to the thought that nothing can prevent deterioration. It may be that this view has affected our practices by steering us away from seeking quality care and relationships which value the individual and demonstrate respect. It may therefore be valuable to seek ways to identify these thoughts and prevent them determining a course of action stemming from the belief that 'nothing can be done'.

An understanding of dementia as a disease or organic impairment is useful to give an insight into the way medical practitioners approach the condition and to understand some of the processes involved, but it adds little to our knowledge for practice. When we come to consider characteristics and clinical features, we are able to see the impact of this underlying pathology and to make connections that may enhance our approach to people and the interventions and services we provide. The importance of interdisciplinary communication cannot be stressed enough.

Characteristics and clinical features

The clinical picture generally described is an impoverishment of memory, both short-term and long-term – including encoding information, storage, retrieval and recollection (Jorm, 1987). A change may be evident in personality and mood. Hallucinations and delusions may also occur. The picture is, to a large extent, determined by the personality of the individual before the onset of the dementia (see Figure 1.3).

Pre-morbid personality

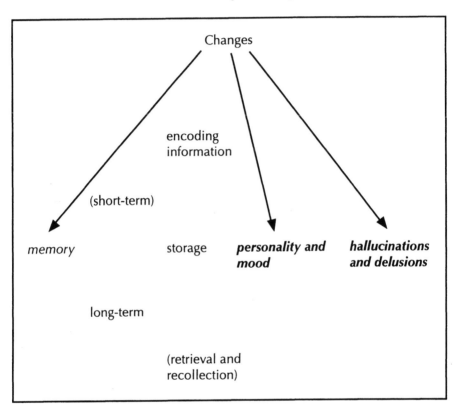

Figure 1.3   Clinical features of dementia

The primary medical descriptions are contained in Lishman (1987) and Gelder et al. (1989). The main points are summarised in Box 1.1.

Box 1.1   Clinical description of dementia

- **Behaviour** becomes disorganised and often inappropriate
- **Thinking** is slowed and impoverished
- **Speech** quality is lost, and meaningless noises are common
- **Mood** in the early stages is often characterised by anxiety and depression, and may change quickly or be blunted in the latter stages
- **Cognitive functioning** is impaired, new learning is difficult, and insight is usually lacking as to the degree and nature of the disorder.

A clear and simple description of the changes occurring in dementia is provided by Lodge (1988) (see Box 1.2).

Box 1.2   The main changes associated with dementia

- **Memory**: Assimilation of information and its retention is difficult, short-term memory is affected, and recent events are often quickly forgotten
- **Orientation**: The sense of time, place, and often the person, is disrupted
- **Grasp**: Making sense of what is happening, judgment and problem-solving is impaired
- **Communication**: Speech deteriorates
- **Personality**: Exaggerated or muted reactions may be noted
- **Behaviour**: Incontinence, wandering, noisiness, aggression may occur
- **Monitoring**: Self-monitoring is neglected
- **Reactions to disease**: These are specific to the individual; mood changes may be noted
- **State**: Whether it is reversible or not
- **Neurology**: Focal damage can cause additional problems.

The characteristics described in Box 1.2 are general, and each individual displays different sets and with different emphases. This depends on the past history and functioning of individuals, where they live and with whom, and what type of disease is thought to cause their dementia. Before we turn to the underlying causes of dementia, you should attempt Activity 1.2.

Activity 1.2

Bearing in mind the characteristics noted in the medical descriptions, think of a person suffering from dementia that you know or have worked with. Construct a profile of that person in terms of these descriptions. What applications might this have in your work with that person?

Comments

Many of us working with people with dementia will be able to think of individuals who forget names, people's faces, where they were or the time of day. We will have memories of people struggling to make themselves understood and becoming frustrated. We will have amusing and heartening reflections as well as sad and upsetting ones. However, it is important to remember that our experiences affect the way we approach these people, and we must constantly reflect on our understandings.

Types of disease causing dementia

There are differences between the many types of disease that underlie or cause dementia. In medical parlance, *nosology* refers to the system by which diseases are classified. We will now consider the following:

- Alzheimer's disease
- multi-infarct dementia
- Pick's disease
- Huntington's disease
- Creutzfeldt-Jakob disease
- Korsakoff's syndrome
- Parkinson's disease
- AIDS.

The most common cause of dementia is *Alzheimer's disease*. This term covers many distinct types of dementia, and in popular understanding it is often used as a blanket term describing dementia. Dementia of the Alzheimer's type has specific characteristics, however.

Clinical examination may reveal impairment of memory and cognitive function at first, and as these changes progress it becomes harder for the person and those around to deny other manifestations of deterioration, including personality changes, increased irritability, anti-social acts, depression and a range of other changes.

The most clearly and commonly recognised problems reported occur in memory, orientation and grasp. A person may forget the names of close relatives, lose his or her way home from the shops, or fail to take in simple instructions to meet a friend for coffee.

CASE STUDY 1.1: LUCY

Lucy Abel had four grandchildren. They came to see her regularly. Recently, however, she had forgotten their names and had not sent a birthday card to her eldest grandchild, Tom, aged 13. When this was mentioned by Tom's mother, Lucy became quite angry and complained that she had too much to remember and that too much was expected of her. She burst into tears and told her daughter how worried and confused she was about what had happened.

In the later stages further neurological changes occur, leading to postural and gait problems, incontinence, focal weaknesses, abnormal reflexes, dysphasia (difficulties in using language), dyspraxia (difficulties in carrying out voluntary actions or movements) and convulsions.

CASE STUDY 1.2: LUCY

As time went on, Lucy found it increasingly difficult to dress in the morning. She was often found with two or more cardigans on, and often the wrong way round. From time to time when talking she would slur her words, or screw up her face tightly when she could not think of the right word to use. When walking she seemed to stoop more and shuffled in small but fairly quick steps.

The pathology of Alzheimer's disease usually shows a progressive and gradual course, during which the brain atrophies, ventricles become enlarged and brain weight decreases. Certain *histopathological features* (those associated with tissue damage) are characteristic. Those mentioned most frequently are the development of *senile plaques* and *neurofibrillary tangles*. Senile plaques are collections of damaged neurons (nerve cells) in the brain. They lead to a scarring of the brain tissue which is evident on examination at post-mortem. Neurofibrillary tangles are twisted filaments of protein found in the neurons throughout the cerebral cortex but especially in the hippocampal region associated with memory. There is also believed to be an increased *nerve cell loss*, especially in the hippocampal region, although it is recognised that the normal ageing brain shows some of the same neuro-pathological changes. At post-mortem examination there appears to be a marked reduction in *choline acetyl transferase* – the enzyme responsible for synthesis of acetylcholine: the neurotransmitter with primary responsibility for the higher mental functions of the brain. Other less marked changes also occur.

These and other changes can be determined by complex investigations using computerised tomography, magnetic resonance imaging and at post-mortem examination. It is important to have a grasp of the basic pathological degeneration, but the clinical picture is of greater relevance in social work.

The second largest cause of dementia is known as *multi-infarct dementia*. It results from cerebrovascular disease of thrombotic, embotic or haemorrhagic nature. In this type of dementia there is usually a sudden deterioration in mental performance. Physically, there is often a corresponding episode of hemiparesis or lack of sensation to one side of the body.

Deterioration in multi-infarct dementia is step-wise, and after an infarct a person may regain most of their functioning or at least show no further deterioration for a time. There is a fluctuation of mental state, a lability (instability) in mood, and the possibility of localised manifestations associated with the damaged site. These may include physical difficulties with limbs or to one side of the body, dysphasia (difficulties with speech) and unilateral weaknesses. Other characteristic changes may include:

- gait and posture
- the display of primitive reflexes – grasping, sucking, and rooting
- oro-facial dyskinesias – involuntary and repetitive movements of the mouth and face
- ideational, ideomotor and motor apraxias – difficulties in perception undertaking actions and co-ordinating them.

Profound changes in behaviour may also result. The emotional changes associated with memory loss and dementia can be compounded by the difficult physical changes that may also occur.

CASE STUDY 1.3: BEATTIE

Beattie James lived on her own and was visited by her son each day. He found her in the hallway, slumped against the wall one day. When he asked her what had happened, she could not remember. What was worse for her at the time was that she could not speak. All that came out was a garbled mass of sounds.

Beattie recovered well from the physical effects of her stroke. Unfortunately, it left her with great difficulty finding the words to say. She became very frustrated by this. She could understand what was said to or asked of her, but could not always reply. She became quite tearful and depressed by these changes.

Other diseases causing dementia

Pick's disease was first described in 1892. It is an inherited condition characterised by a marked degeneration of the frontal and temporal lobes in particular, and a lesser degree of general atrophy. Clinical symptoms reflect the site of the damage. Initially, deterioration in personality and mood disorders are often more apparent than memory and language problems. Having said this, differential diagnosis is difficult to make as the progress is similar to that of Alzheimer's disease. Often it is not until autopsy that a firm diagnosis is given. Pick's disease can appear at any age, but is most common between the ages of 50 and 60, and women are twice as likely to be affected as men (Gelder et al., 1989; Lishman, 1987; Wilcock, 1990).

Huntington's disease was described by a New England physician, George Huntington, in 1872. Again, it is an inherited condition. Most damage to the brain occurs in the deep-lying areas of grey matter. The age of onset is fairly young, usually between 25 and 50 years. At first, neurological signs are most noticeable, and psychiatric symptoms occur somewhat later. Early signs are choreiform movements of face, hands and shoulders (sudden unexpected, aimless and forceful movements). These progress to a point at which walking, eating and sitting become difficult or impossible. Memory is less affected, and insight can remain until fairly late. Not surprisingly, perhaps, apathy and depression are common. When cognitive impairment does occur, it is often focal and progresses quite slowly.

Creutzfeldt-Jakob disease was described independently by two physicians, Creutzfeldt in 1920 and Jakob in 1921. It is a rapidly progressing degenerative disease of the nervous system characterised by intellectual deterioration and various neurological deficits.

A variant of the disease has been likened to a human form of bovine spongiform encephalopathy (more popularly referred to as 'mad cow disease'). There is evidence that it is transmissible and is caused by a slow-acting virus, but it is a fairly rare disease.

Chronic and heavy use of *alcohol* is associated, as a contributory cause, with the development of dementia. This is sometimes linked to a thiamine deficiency and to *Korsakoff's syndrome* or *Korsakoff's psychosis*. Memory and intellectual functioning can be permanently impaired, although slight improvement, or at least no further deterioration, can result from abstinence.

Cerebral atrophy that is assumed to give rise to the symptoms of disorientation, confusion and memory loss has been observed for many years in chronic alcohol abuse, although in cases of severe and progressive dementia there may be coincident Alzheimer's disease (Lishman, 1987).

Some people suffering from *Parkinson's disease* also show intellectual impairment, though not the majority. There appears to be a greater association with people suffering from 'arteriosclerotic parkinsonism', which may suggest a link with cerebral arteriosclerosis (a hardening of the arteries). However, some cases of cognitive decline have also occurred in people with idiopathic Parkinson's. The prevalence of senile plaques and tangles suggests that a pathology similar to Alzheimer's disease is present in some people.

AIDS is particularly important to the present discussion. A wide range of symptoms are seen, including personality change, memory disorder, confusion, ataxia and focal neurological signs.

It has been estimated that up to 90 per cent of people suffering from AIDS have neuropathological evidence of central nervous system abnormalities. It appears that HIV is in some way linked to the development of a dementia. Of that 90 per cent, about half show evidence of a clinical dementia by death.

Whilst it is clear that dementia is most often associated with increasing age, this brief exploration of diseases underlying dementia demonstrates that it can occur at various stages throughout a person's life. It is important to bear this in mind because of the tendency to assume that old age and memory impairment or deterioration in functioning are necessarily linked.

Summary

The medical definition and description of dementia holds sway not only over the medical profession, but is also accepted by nursing professionals (Jones and Miesen, 1992), social policy theorists (Norman, 1982), psychologists (Bromley, 1988), and social work and social care professionals (Marshall, 1990; Harvey, 1990). However, the medical understanding describes a disease process that, as we noted earlier, is different for each individual, depending upon their life experiences, coping skills, functioning, living situation, beliefs and values, and physical constitution, among other factors. Also, the medical description itself is often unclear. Murphy (1986) states:

It is not always straightforward to tell one form of dementia from another, especially when someone has been suffering from the condition for a few years.

But medical researchers can tell from looking at the brain after death which illness the patient was suffering. At present the distinction ... is not really helpful in treatment, but it is helpful in research, and research will eventually lead to our overcoming this group of diseases. (p. 18)

The medical model provides a linear understanding which suggests that, given the right treatment, a cure is possible. This is perhaps not surprising, but it is important to remember that individuals with specific and particular needs are involved. Ways of approaching, understanding and accepting and managing the disease need to be worked upon before reaching for the dream of a cure which remains elusive. We shall now turn to some of the ways sociologists have approached and explained dementia.

Sociological approaches to dementia

From the famous sociological study of suicide by Durkheim at the end of the nineteenth century, sociology has shown an interest in mental health. Sociological approaches to mental ill health also include discussions of dementia. In this section we will review three major sociological approaches to dementia:

- structural approaches
- interactionist approaches
- ethnomethodological approaches.

Mental illness is viewed by *structuralists* (who believe that an individual's behaviour is dependent upon their social environment and the prescriptions and prohibitions of that society) as the result of particular aspects of their social structure, such as class, gender, age and race (Bond, 1987). Dementia could be seen as part of a response to changing roles in society, and as an adaptive process of disengagement from social activities as the individual ages. This view implies that dementia is part of 'normal' ageing. Withdrawal from social roles and a rationalisation of inequalities in power and status by virtue of age are also implied in the structuralist view. This view was popular in the 1960s but is criticised as giving credence to the claims of ageism in associating age with deterioration, decline and withdrawal (Cumming and Henry, 1961).

Interactionist sociologists take a different view. Mental illness is not thought to be clearly defined, but is viewed as a social status conferred upon a person by other members of that society, usually on the basis of a judgement about the individual's behaviour. It is dependent on social interaction in which a label is applied – in this case, dementia – and future behaviour towards that person takes place in the context of that label.

Activity 1.3

Return briefly to Activity 1.2. You may find instances in which labels have been applied to people with dementia. You may also be able to think of times in which your perceptions have been confirmed or challenged by direct contact and communication with people with dementia. Spend a little time considering the implications for your practice.

This approach differs from the structuralist approach because individuals have to make sense, interpret and give meaning to their world, rather than the world outside exerting a governing control. People take an active part in creating their own roles. As we have already seen, one of the reasons the Royal College of Physicians (1981) provided their operational definition of dementia was to counteract the prevailing view within the medical profession that ageing and dementia could be considered as almost synonymous.

Some people have greater power to ascribe labels (Szasz, 1971; Parker and Randall 1997a). In the area of mental illness it is psychiatrists who categorise and apply labels that define a person as mentally ill. The categories are not accepted automatically, and disagreements occur over the interpretation and meanings given to observed behaviours. Differentiating people as 'mentally ill' and 'normal' may be contingent upon the particular circumstances of the social situation in which people find themselves.

The individual's interpretation and the meaning they give to their own actions and those of others are important to interactionists (Bond et al., 1990).

The *ethnomethodological* approach is similar to the interactionist view. It assumes a continual creation of the social world by its members. People use a 'taken-for-granted' knowledge about how the world operates and how they can deal with it in ways acceptable to them.

Rather than study mental illness as a discrete entity, ethnomethodologists would consider the way societies build concepts of relevance in understanding mental illness. An example would be the biographical approach to Alzheimer's disease. In this approach the construction of diverse biographies by people around an individual is seen to have practical value in producing a descriptive biography of an individual. The social processes involved in the production and reproduction of biographies is important to the ethnomethodologist (Gubrium and Lynott, 1985; Gubrium, 1986). Alzheimer's disease is not itself the focus, but is used as a code for informing us about how the resulting difficulties are understood and lived with in society.

These sociological approaches to dementia do not deny the validity of the medical models developed. They add to the way people suffering from dementia may be understood and seen as individual agents in a wide and varied living environment.

Scrutton (1989) points out that there is no single agreed cause or definition of dementia, and certainly none proven. As noted above when describing the medical models, the links between the neuropathology and dementia are inconsistent. Also, there are flashes of lucidity and non-confused behaviour in people labelled as having dementia.

Many of the approaches deriving from sociology see mental illness as a judgement made about an individual's or group's deviation from 'normal' or more socially acceptable behaviour (Goffman, 1961; Scheff, 1966; Szasz, 1974). However, there are a number of complex social and environmental factors involved, and confused behaviour can be seen as a coded but meaningful communication about the problems of living (Meacher, 1972; Scrutton, 1989).

Social trauma is also linked to biochemical and hormonal changes that lead to psychological disturbances such as depression (see Claridge, 1986; Goldberg and Huxley, 1992; Brown and Harris, 1978). The stress arising from social perceptions of ageing and worth may have such an impact on a person to lead to confusion and withdrawal from the world. A well-established response to stress is to withdraw, to feel sorry for oneself, to become anti-social. In older people that label of confusion has been used to explain this withdrawal. Whereas early structuralists interpreted withdrawal as a natural process, its links to psychosocial stress demonstrate the potentially negative effects of society on the functioning of individuals, and emphasise the power of labelling others.

Isolation often plays an additional part. Lack of communication with others and a lack of understanding from others contribute, as does growing dependence and fear.

CASE STUDY 1.4: EDWARD

Edward Breakwell had been a regular supporter of his local rugby team. He had a position on the supporters' club and was instrumental in bringing local schools to the ground. Over the last three years, since his wife died, he had become less active in the club. In fact, no one had seen him for three or four months. This worried some of his long-standing acquaintances.

Two men from the supporters' club went to visit Edward and to see if they could bring him back. They were shocked by the reception they received. At first Edward sat huddled in a chair and hardly spoke to them. He then said he wanted nothing to do with the club, got up and walked out of the house, telling his visitors to lock up when they wanted to leave. They vowed never to see 'that ungrateful bugger' again.

The psychosocial understanding of dementia has taken up these issues and, after Activity 1.4, we shall turn to this.

Activity 1.4

Return again to your initial description and definition of dementia, and to the description of someone you know or have worked with. Can you identify any of the events, thoughts or characteristics mentioned above in relation to that person? How might this affect your understanding of dementia and your approach to people suffering from dementia?

Comments

The original descriptions you made may have been constructed in the light of your experience of dementia, older people and your local and cultural background. These understandings will lead to certain judgements and, if accepted uncritically, will place people into boxes without seeing the individual. As humans, we continuously create and re-create our world and understanding of it, but we need to be aware of this process and to use it as a basis for understanding rather than categorising people.

A psychosocial approach to dementia

One particularly useful contribution to understanding dementia comes from the work of Tom Kitwood and his associates at the Bradford Dementia Research Group. From his early research into dementia (Kitwood, 1988), he began to see psychosocial stress as a possible contributory factor to the development of dementia. He considered a range of evidence from post-mortem studies that indicated considerable variation in neuropathology. He gathered evidence suggesting that some people who displayed the clinical symptoms of dementia had very little neurological damage. Some people who displayed severe brain damage at autopsy had remained mentally intact. Thus he concluded that the links between neuropathology and dementia are loose and by no means entirely proven.

Kitwood (1988) developed an understanding that considers the whole person. By using social and cognitive psychology, he described how self-concept arises from social feedback and social comparison. This is similar to the sociological approaches reviewed. In the most healthy settings, people are valued and respected. This leads to a positive self-image. Where this positive sense of self is removed, as occurs in dementia, the sense of being or identity is lost. Kitwood, like Scrutton (1989), proposes the concept of the *dementogenic social environment*. This means that the context in which the individual lives bears responsibility for much of the characteristic deterioration and decline associated with people suffering from dementia.

Kitwood (1990) developed these ideas further. He argued that there are difficulties in seeing a linear causal relationship between brain pathology and dementia, and therefore suggested that dementia arises from a combination of negative social reactions and neurological impairment. Neurological impairment attracts a negative response or *malignant social psychology*. Because the physiological buffers of the person are weakened, this can create further neurological impairment. His ideas are tentative, but he provides a useful list of processes and interactions that depersonalise the person with dementia – what he calls 'malignant social psychology'(see Box 1.3).

Box 1.3   Kitwood's malignant social psychology

- treachery – dishonest representation and trickery
- disempowerment – things done for and to a person
- infantilisation – extreme disempowerment
- intimidation – by professional involvement
- labelling – leads to different treatment because of the label
- stigmatisation – like labelling, but including exclusion
- outpacing – carers carry on at normal speed, leaving the sufferer behind
- invalidation – subjectivity and experiences of the sufferer are ignored
- banishment – deprivation of human contact because of the dementia
- objectification – the person is not treated as such, but as an impersonal object.

Activity 1.5

Think of malignant social psychology, as described in Box 1.3, and identify some of the factors in your work situation and in your practice. Consider ways in which you can acknowledge your approach and develop ways of working that validate individual traits and needs.

Kitwood (1990) then suggests four reasons why neurological impairment attracts such interactions:

1   There is a lack of insight into the person's present experiences of life.
2   The pressure and 'busyness' of caretaking can wear down carers.
3   There is a tendency not to treat the person as a valuable or sentient being.
4   Anxieties and fears about our own possible futures may lead to avoidance of contact with the sufferer.

His model proposes that losses and changes in early later life – from the sixth decade onwards – impose a great strain on the psyche. If adequate adjustment can be made, all well and good. If not, however, the person is left in a particularly vulnerable state. If a significant loss of brain tissue occurs, a progressive process of dementia, with the attraction of malignant social psychology, may result.

This is similar to the approach taken by two other psychologists, Riordan and Whitmore (1990). They suggest from wide experience that:

• The person is *aware* of being confused, and of the *fear* this creates
• Their *sense of control* over external and internal events is limited and vulnerable
• They develop a *sense of helplessness*, believing they have little or no power to influence their world
• *Denial* may be common because of the pain involved in admitting to confusion.

They present an optimistic view with which to approach dementia that questions the usefulness of labelling, and allows a constructive approach to develop, aimed at change and enhancement of the quality of life. Their view is that social learning does continue, but it continues in a negative and debilitating way. The person is ascribed a label that, to them and others, implies a lack or failure of competence. The activity is taken over by another person, thus removing opportunities for practice, incentive and reward. This leads to inability and helplessness.

Gilleard (1984) accepts that whilst an understanding of the underlying neuropathologies is important, it is more important to consider what constitutes the self, and what gives a person integrity, consistency and value. Thus Gilleard describes dementia by reference to the observed symptoms and behaviours (see Box 1.4).

Box 1.4   Common changes in people with dementia

Cognitive changes: these are usually characterised by failures of retrieval and storage of information, and focal deficits such as expression of speech, writing and spatial and bodily orientation. Problem-solving and abstract conceptual reasoning is impaired.

Emotional changes: these can involve extreme anxiety and agitation or emotional flatness.

Behavioural changes:

- wandering and restlessness in terms of habitual behaviour, stalking old haunts, or disorientation and inability to sustain goal-directed actions
- incontinence, which may be the result of localised physical or psychological reasons such as infection, depression, or the indirect consequence of mobility problems, dressing problems, or a loss of learned bladder control
- aggression and hostility may be displayed as a disinhibited over-reaction and frustration, a misinterpretation of events or a defensive reaction.

Of course, these behavioural manifestations lend themselves to an approach that is concerned with changing and modifying patterns of expressed behaviour. A challenge to this would be that new learning is impaired. However, not only is behaviour experienced and expressed in a social context, but each individual has a different potential for experience and a different level of awareness.

Kitwood (1990) and Kitwood and Bredin (1992) designed an approach to the evaluation of dementia care based upon these ideas. They suggest that by respecting the personhood of the sufferer and demonstrating their relative well-being, the person's quality of life can be enhanced and extended.

This approach does not deny that damage to the brain is important, but adds that the deterioration and impairment is affected by the interactions to people in conjunction with the pathology. This places dementia in a social, interactive context and gives a place to the perceptions and values of individuals involved. Behavioural approaches which acknowledge the systemic, interactive context of living fit well with this approach. Kitwood (1997a, 1997b) describes the new culture in terms of personhood. He suggests the following criteria for the model:

- Categories used to describe people with dementia should be equally applicable to practitioners using them
- People are acknowledged to be social and interactive beings
- People can change for good or ill throughout their lives
- People are different psychologically, physically and neurologically
- Best practice should be pursued to meet people's needs.

CASE STUDY 1.5: MARTHA

Martha Williams lived in Bay Tree House, a local authority residential care home. She had lived there for two years. Throughout that time, staff reported a steady and significant decline in what she could do for herself and in her communication. She received no visits from her family. Martha was left to herself. She was quiet and undemanding, never being known to object to bathing, dressing or going to bed, and never making a complaint, but she was lethargic and apathetic. This was considered to be part of her dementia, and staff were pleased she was so compliant.

A change of management brought with it new practices. These were at first resisted as unnecessary and time-consuming without leading to gains. The manager wanted individual time to be spent with each person, to find out their wants and wishes and to make them feel wanted. Martha remained uncommunicative, but the manager herself pointed to the way she looked at her keyworker and the small curl in her lips that was almost a smile.

Summary

The medical, sociological and psychological approaches to dementia need not be seen as mutually exclusive. In fact, it is best to see them as interdependent. Whilst the diseases underlying the personal and mental deterioration are important and may in the future provide means and methods of retarding its progress and treating the person, it is equally important to consider how the disease and its characteristics are interpreted by the sufferer, carer, professionals and wider society. These understandings have a great bearing upon the approaches to intervention undertaken, and, in a wider sense, the policies and care provided. In the final section to this chapter we will consider the context and location of social work practice where dementia is an issue.

Activity 1.6

Make a list of the main features of the medical model, sociological models and the psychosocial approach. Which do you think is most valuable for your work with people with dementia?

Identify some of the links between the approaches, and consider how this knowledge might help you in your practice.

Social work and dementia

Social workers practise in the context of care management, which is the subject of Chapter 2. Within these organisational settings, however, social workers play a number of roles and use a wide range of strategies to provide high-quality and consistent care to people suffering from dementia. Many of these approaches are necessarily concerned with the provision of effective practical care and support. Others relate to interventive techniques and strategies designed to improve and enhance people's quality of life in respectful ways. These comprise:

- behaviour, task and action-focused techniques
- counselling and psychotherapeutic techniques
- group, community and social approaches.

Part II of this book provides a systematic review and consideration of the main methods and approaches which can be used with people with dementia and their carers. These are also transferable to other areas of practice.

Social work with people with dementia and their carers is indebted to the work of Mary Marshall and her colleagues at the Dementia Services Development Centre in Stirling, and to the pioneering work of Tom Kitwood and his team at the Bradford Dementia Research Group. From a time less than two decades ago when working with people with dementia was marginalised and almost sneered at, we have in many ways entered the exciting time of a 'new culture of care' (Kitwood and Benson, 1995).

The new culture of dementia care actively promotes respect for people with dementia and their carers. It stresses the 'personhood' of these individuals – it views people first as valuable, unique individuals with their own history, experiences, wants and wishes. It is therefore important to view dementia from an integrated perspective, acknowledging that the individual, his or her past and present characteristics, likes and dislikes, is as important as the medical condition or disease underlying the changes.

None of the books addressing dementia care provides a systematic review of interventive strategies, techniques and their uses and limitations with people with dementia and their carers, although many provide a wide range of useful and important strategies. Jones and Miesen (1992) provide a comprehensive edited collection which reviews a number of models and theories for dementia care and an array of interventions for use in residen-- tial settings, in the community and within families. Descriptions and analyses of interventions are included concerning:

- reality orientation
- reminiscence and life review
- validation work
- music therapy
- psychotherapy
- carers' groups
- care services.

Their work does not deal with the practical implementation of these strategies. On the positive side, it emphasises the importance of interdisciplinary work in providing high-quality care services to people with dementia and their carers.

Very few practice-related texts are intended solely for social work audiences. In part this reflects the necessity of an interdisciplinary approach and the value of the whole person. However, interest in working with older people and a shift in the perceived value of the work came about after publication of Marshall's *Social Work with Old People* (Marshall, 1983) and with Froggatt's *Family Work with Elderly People* (Froggatt, 1990). Although these books did not relate solely to dementia, they added to the knowledge of and skills for social work practice in these areas. In 1993, however, Chapman and Marshall published a text directed at social workers and their practice skills in working with people with dementia and their carers. The book responded to a growing need for a practice guide, an increasing recognition of the importance of the work, and a valuing of the uniqueness and worth of individuals with dementia and their carers. This book was timely and a landmark in social work practice, but it did not address all skills and practice methods of use with people with dementia, restricting itself to a discussion of psychotherapy, reminiscence, family therapy, groupwork and empowerment.

Prior to this, Marshall (1990) published an edited practice guide. This brought an important array of knowledge in an accessible form to a variety of professionals working in this area, but it provided little in terms of direct intervention methods. In the chapter on this subject, the emphasis lay predominantly on dealing with difficult behaviours and problems and creating the best residential environment.

At the same time that this work was developing in the field of social and health care practice, Kitwood and Bredin (1992) published another guide that emphasised the individual worth of people with dementia. Whilst intended to provide practical advice on the care of people with dementia, it set the foundations for a value base for that care: it emphasised 'personhood'. This emphasis on values was repeated by Chapman et al. (1994) in their book for day and residential care staff. They stress the five principles of care developed by the King's Fund:

1 People with dementia have the same human value as anyone else, irrespective of their degree of disability or independence.
2 People with dementia have the same varied human needs as anyone else.
3 People with dementia have the same rights as other citizens.
4 Every person with dementia is an individual.
5 People with dementia have the right to forms of support that do not exploit families or friends.

They use this value base to describe good therapeutic care, and suggest that a sound knowledge of each individual is essential to planning intervention. This may be gained by life-story work. The interventions will differ from person to person but will be built around the following general principles:

• maintaining a focus on retained abilities
• providing adequate stimulation, including physical activity, conversation, crafts, games, daily chores, singing dancing and reminiscing

- sensitive prompting.

The practice strategies reviewed briefly in this book include:

- reality orientation
- reminiscence
- validation
- listening and responding
- diversion
- behaviour therapy.

There has been a spate of recent books dealing with people with dementia. Marshall (1996) writes for all involved in contemporary health and social care of people with dementia. The emphasis on values and a new, developing culture which celebrates uniqueness is retained. Whilst a good deal of the book concerns the organisational and legislative context of health and social care, there is a chapter on interventions. She terms this 'therapy', but agrees the word is odd in this context. Therapy is, for Marshall, the reduction of anguish and pain. The book outlines strategies from behaviour management, social and physical activities, counselling, groupwork and family therapy. Marshall (1997) includes many useful chapters on a broad range of themes, but little concerning direct practice.

Goldsmith (1996) considers the perspective of the person with dementia and encourages practitioners to listen to the person's story and to examine their own perceptions and views of dementia and its meanings. The edited collection by Hunter (1997) provides an up-to-date and refreshing look at the 'new culture', including chapters on social work, social care, psychology and psychiatry. It does not provide a detailed account of methods for practice but sets out a clear alternative framework for understanding dementia and advocates strongly for an increased awareness of and emphasis on communication and listening both for people with dementia and their carers.

Part II of this book will introduce a wide range of direct practice methods which can ground the new approaches to dementia care, promote and enable people's choice, and increase dignity and respect.

2 The context of care management

Introduction

The introduction of the National Health Service and Community Care Act 1990 has brought with it fundamental changes to the process and organisation of social services in general. This is no less the case for people with dementia. Of course, the move towards 'community care', however that may be defined, has a long history. Whilst in its present form it can be traced back at least to the Percy Commission reporting on mental health law prior to the passing and implementation of the Mental Health Act 1959 (Percy Report, 1957), there has been an official policy of care in the community of some description since the days of the Poor Law. The nineteenth century saw an increase in the development of institutions and segregation of those labelled as deviant, including people with mental health problems and many older people, but this development was not total.

This chapter will review the development of the present concept of community care and some of the characteristics of care management as the context for social work and social care work with people who have dementia.

The development of modern community care policies

After the construction of the welfare state, the passing of the National Assistance Act 1948, National Health Service Act 1946, and the implementation of the Mental Health Act 1959, a mood of optimism prevailed. Attitudes towards people with mental health problems became more tolerant.

Drug treatments appeared to offer cure or management to people with long-term mental health conditions. A corresponding and general concern for civil rights grew, especially in the light of a number of inquiries into bad practice in institutions (DHSS, 1969, 1971, 1972). In this context, and alongside a changing society in demographic terms and in terms of composition of and attitude towards family and community, a concern to re-establish people in their own local, familiar and chosen environments developed. In 1962, the Minister for Health, Enoch Powell, presented his blueprint for the hospitals, which involved the closure of long-stay psychiatric units and the establishment of care in local, accessible units within the community (Ministry of Health, 1962). Matters did not proceed as intended, and despite the efforts of policymakers and concerned individuals throughout social and health care, the numbers remained high in institutional settings. Also, the optimism of earlier years changed with the realisation that physical treatments for mental health problems had side-effects and potentially damaging implications, and often only limited success, people became concerned about implications for jobs, and there was a developing sense of cost and resource implications within care settings. Thus progress was slow.

Concern for costs of welfare and social and health care grew as changes in the world markets and in economic thought filtered down. The growth of 'New Right' thinking, epitomised by Margaret Thatcher's governments of the late 1970s and throughout the 1980s, emphasised efficiency in costs and finding the most effective solutions at the cheapest cost.

Underpinning the legislation concerning community care are a number of assumptions and beliefs about the nature of welfare which apply to both ends of the political spectrum. It is due to the fact that the concept of community care is located within the wider framework of these differing political views that there is some apparent divergence in responses to the concept in practice. It is also useful to discuss some of the political and economic pressures in order to provide an appropriate context for the concept.

Throughout the past three decades, the pressures faced by administrations of both Labour and Conservative governments have been increasing. Growth in the total public expenditure had been experienced by all Western countries since the 1950s (Leat, 1986) but was slowing down by the late 1970s. The relative increase in the number of economically dependent people in relation to those who were economically productive began to produce arguments about the 'burdens of dependency'. From the late 1970s, a policy of retrenchment was apparent. Crossland's famous statement, 'the party's over,' heralded the publication of the Labour document *Priorities for Health and Social Services* (DHSS, 1976), and this was followed by a Conservative publication *Care in Action* (DHSS, 1981a). Both documents gave overt and explicit recognition to a need to identify priorities in expenditure and to manage limited resources for health and welfare within existing budgets. There was a clear statement that the expenditure on social welfare must be preceded by the adequate production of economic wealth.

From 1979, however, the economic policies of the Conservative government became more radical. These policies sought ultimately to reformulate the parameters of state responsibility and the terms on which distribution of the provision of welfare should be premised. The justification for these political concepts and assumptions was derived principally from such market theorists as Hayek (1960) and Friedman and Friedman (1980). The thinking of this 'New Right' tapped a groundswell of concern about the efficiency and effectiveness of state welfare provision. The implications drawn from such thinking were clearly that large-scale provision of welfare support for individuals created and fostered a culture of dependency which was anachronistic in terms of the current society where real incomes for the employed were continuing to rise. In addition to this was the appearance of broader social policies which advocated individualism, self-help and personal responsibility for actions. The speech given by Fowler in 1985 (the so-called 'Buxton Speech', see McCarthy, 1990) encapsulated the predominant political ethos of that time with the promotion of private and voluntary provision of care for those in need in a new 'mixed economy' of welfare. The prevailing ideology can also be seen in such statements as: 'Community care means care by the community' (DHSS, 1981b).

At the same time as this shift in political and economic thought was taking place, the field of social welfare was seeing the development of concepts concerning de-institutionalisation. The restrictive and dehumanising effects of institutions (in particular those concerned with mental health) had been recognised and documented (Laing, 1965; Goffman, 1961). In addition, from the early 1980s an increasing number of publications had been documenting the ineffectiveness of public sector provision of welfare (Hadley and Hatch, 1981; Barclay Report, 1982; Audit Commission, 1986; King's Fund, 1987; Griffiths Report, 1988). Such writings argued for the creation of a pluralist system of welfare.

The Wagner Report published in 1988 added a further complexity to the field by highlighting the problems arising from public funding of private residential care and the apparently perverse incentives available to older people to enter residential care and obtain assistance with funding. From the early 1980s there had been a shift in emphasis from the traditional view – that only people with means could afford to enter private care – to provision by the DHSS of payments towards the cost of such care. This had resulted in a rapid increase in the number of people exercising their right to choose care and to enter private care homes, which in turn had led to an escalating bill for the government running into millions of pounds of payments via the DHSS for care (and a need to control this) and suspicions on the part of the government that the vast majority of elderly people entering private homes did not require that level of care, because eligibility for DHSS assistance was based on income, with no assessment of care needs. This latter view was not borne out by research, however (see Allen et al., 1992, for further exposition).

These aspects were picked up again in the Griffiths Report (1988), which discussed the need to assist people to remain living at home and to set up a new system for funding of private residential care from the public purse. The development of real alternatives to institutional care was expounded, together with exhortations that government policies and state provision of welfare should move away from resource and service-led provision to needs-led provision, and that individuals and their carers should be offered more choice of provision. Yet a further argument developed from the Canadian-based 'service brokerage' model of case management, in which a shift from the provision of standardised types of care to more individualised services was advocated. Furthermore, within such systems, client advocacy and user control of service provision was seen as the way forward (Salisbury, 1989; Brandon, 1989).

Community care, care management and needs-led assessment have a variety of different meanings for different people. This can be seen not just in the public/professional interface, but also at the interdisciplinary level. To expand slightly, the political Right appear to have developed the concepts to fit with the perception of low-cost solutions to social problems' (care in the community being seen consistently as a lower-cost option than residential care). Within this type of model, the development of private forms of welfare is welcomed and the responsibility of the state for collective provision of welfare is marginalized and residualized. On the other hand, the political Left has viewed such concepts as an opportunity to promote user empowerment and also to demystify the professionalisation of welfare systems (and in particular, professional assessments of individuals). Although such views are polarised and have been somewhat exaggerated in order to emphasise the extent of the continuum, elements of each type of view appear in the current publications pertaining to needs-led assessment. The degree to which the ideal is achievable depends partly on the ideological and political stance of the particular author, and also on their own interpretation of policy.

The Audit Commission (1986) also indicated that proposed community care initiatives from the last two decades were not being realised. The government therefore asked Sir Roy Griffiths to report on possibilities for speeding up the process and how business principles could be applied to this area. The Griffiths Report (1988) proposed the germ of the present concept of community care. Although local authorities were to retain their organising function, the report also suggested a move towards design and purchasing of services rather than direct service provision. These ideas were quickly translated into a White Paper, *Caring for People*, (DoH, 1989) and legislation, the National Health Service and Community Care Act 1990.

In many ways contemporary community care policy is little different to the past. However, it positively promotes a commitment to the independence of individuals and to enabling people to reach their full potential.

The White Paper (DoH, 1989) brought the mixed economy of care to centre stage. Local authority social services departments were to have responsibility to ensure that carers were assisted and supported, but the provision of services was to be undertaken by a mix of public sector services and the voluntary and private sectors.

Activity 2.1

What is your understanding of community care? Do you believe it is helpful to the delivery of care services, or do you believe it hinders caregiving? Write down reasons for your thoughts.

Comments

You may believe that care in people's own environments is the best possible option as it validates who they are and their identity. You may recognise some difficulties in practice and in terms of services. It is useful to set the principles of care in the community against those of best dementia care, and to seek ways in which practice can indeed promote choice, rights, dignity and respect, and work with the strengths of individuals.

Some characteristics of community care

Care management is the method of service delivery favoured by the government in setting up, organising and providing community care services (Orme and Glastonbury, 1993). In principle at least, it is about the empowerment of service users. There is a right to assessment enshrined in law (National Health Service and Community Care Act 1990, s. 47), although the eligibility criteria are to a large extent locally determined. The involvement of service users in decisions about services and in monitoring and evaluating the delivery of services is designed to give them greater control.

CASE STUDY 2.1: DAPHNE AND MRS JONES

When Daphne Edwardes requested help for her mother, she thought she would be able to tell the social worker what she thought her mother needed and it would be arranged. She did not see any point in the social worker talking with her mother because she 'constantly forgets things' and 'has no idea she's a risk to herself'. However, after listening intently and actively to what Daphne said, the social worker arranged to see her mother.

Over a short period of four sessions the social worker built a rapport with Daphne's mother, Mrs Jones, and gained her views on support services, which she welcomed as 'taking some of the burden off Daphne'. Daphne was pleasantly surprised.

The *quality assurance* of services delivered is an essential feature of community care. Thus the appropriateness and effectiveness of interventions is an issue whose profile is raised. Related to the development of effective quality assurance is the proposed development of *complaints procedures*. There needs to be a forum which does not just deal with complaints but which can encourage dialogue about the best ways of meeting needs and delivering services. Also important to the care management process is the *monitoring of services* provided, and continuous identification of changing patterns

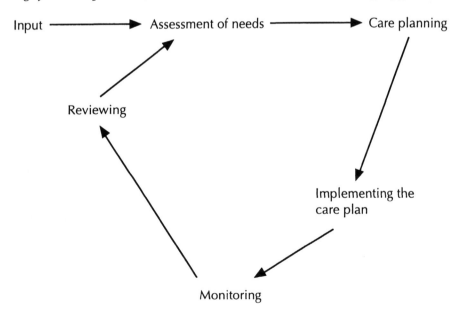

Source: SSI (1992).

Figure 2.1   The care management cycle

of demand. This will, hopefully, provide cost-effective service delivery by planning to meet needs when and where identified, and also aim to account for needs not met elsewhere.

The care management process can be seen as a cycle in which a person's needs are assessed, identified, accounted for, evaluated and reassessed on a regular and continued basis, as shown in Figure 2.1.

It is within this context that social work and social care services for people with dementia are now organised and delivered. The assessment, implementation, and monitoring of these services demand an assurance of their quality and effectiveness with respect to the underlying value base. This dictates that people fare best in their own familiar and chosen environment, and that the services provided are directed towards achieving these objectives.

CASE STUDY 2.2: DAPHNE AND MRS JONES

Mrs Jones was assessed as needing opportunities to enjoy social activities, while maintaining an adequate diet and fluid intake. She did not want her daughter to take responsibility for her, and expressed considerable guilt and anxiety about being 'a burden'.

A plan was discussed and agreed with Mrs Jones and with her daughter, Daphne. This included using Mrs Jones's communication skills to introduce her to a day centre at which she could join in the range of social and informal activities, meeting new people and having a day out of the house. Also, Mrs Jones agreed to a care worker coming to the house to plan with her what she would like to eat that day. She would then encourage Mrs Jones to cook with her.

Daphne had reservations. She hoped that her mother would have been given a range of services, whether or not she wanted them, but agreed to the care. She did feel her views had been listened to. At the first review meeting, which Daphne, Mrs Jones, the social worker, day and home care staff attended, it was agreed by everyone that the care plan had a positive effect in caring for and raising the self-esteem of Mrs Jones. A further benefit was that Daphne felt much more relaxed about her mother's care needs.

Cost implications have also become increasingly important in the provision of services, given resource constraints and drives towards rationalisation and financial savings. Therefore, the need for an effective, ethical and efficient interactive approach is paramount.

Activity 2.2

How are the principles of the care management model of community care promoted and achieved in your work setting?

Make a list of the positive benefits of care management to social care work, and in particular to service users. Make another list outlining some of the difficulties and problems that have resulted.

Comments

Positive benefits listed may include similar ones to those mentioned in relation to Mrs Jones in Case study 2.2. The principles of partnership, joint decisions, respecting rights and promoting dignity are fundamental to the process. There is, of course, an important recognition of the need for protection, and also of the needs of other people involved in each situation.

However, some of the problems result from the needs people have and social workers' determination 'to do a good job'. Priorities need to be set and time needs to be managed.

Each person's work experience will be different, but perhaps the common theme will be one of values for practice.

Older people, dementia and care management

Social workers perform a balancing act between their remit to optimise the social functioning of individuals, families and groups with whom they work, and the legislative framework in which they act as paid employees of a local authority. This is further complicated by the fact that definitions of social functioning and the legislative context are dynamic and continually changing.

Also, social workers have an obligation to be ethical, effective and purposeful in carrying out their duties (BASW, 1975). The goal is to resolve the most pressing problem by focused, directed intervention aimed at helping the client develop new adaptive coping skills.

The more specific social work role with older people is to ensure choice and flexibility of service provision and intervention, and to enable a person to remain in their chosen environment for as long as is practicable. This is especially the case where dementia is an issue, as evidence demonstrates the value of consistency, familiarity and enabling a person to stay within their chosen environment in prolonging orientation and preserving quality of life (Riordan and Whitmore, 1990; Marshall, 1990). In order to accomplish this, the social worker needs to undertake a full and comprehensive assessment of the situation, and to co-ordinate the most appropriate forms of intervention. This accords with the local authority duties as specified in the National Health Service and Community Care Act 1990, in particular sections 46–47.

CASE STUDY 2.3: DAPHNE AND MRS JONES

Mrs Jones's daughter, Daphne, was going on holiday and her usual care worker was off sick. The social worker and Daphne were concerned about Mrs Jones during this period and wanted to ensure she was safe and services were adequate. Daphne's preferred option was short-term respite care. Her mother did not wish to entertain the idea. The social worker suggested a relief care worker and knew she could arrange this, but Mrs Jones did not want a 'stranger' in her house. She suggested an alternative: 'I could go to the day centre each day'. This was a very difficult option for the social worker to arrange, but it was one which was acceptable to all parties and met identified needs. It was arranged.

The fundamental aim of the present community care initiative is to promote independence as far as practicable. In order to optimise service options for users and carers, assessment has been separated from service provision. The concept of care management was introduced as a framework within which these changes could be articulated. Care management aims to co-ordinate services and interventions to ensure that needs are being met in the most appropriate and effective way. The care manager seeks to ensure coherence, to maintain communication and to review. They may be also involved in developing plans, and negotiation with a variety of agencies.

Social workers are obliged to pay attention to the needs of carers too, and to enable them to continue their caring role for as long as is practicable by the provision of practical help, support and advice. This has been enshrined in law in the Carers (Recognition and Services) Act 1995.

CASE STUDY 2.4: DAPHNE AND MRS JONES

Although Daphne's wishes for her mother were not granted, she did feel that she had been listened to and, when services were introduced, she saw that they took her own needs into account. She was pleased with the services. She had heard from friends and neighbours that social services do very little and will not put in help if a relative is supporting the person. She found this to be untrue.

Summary

In this chapter the history and development of community care and care management have been introduced. The care management process and its underlying value base has been discussed, and the case studies have demonstrated how this relates to people with dementia and their carers.

It is in this context that social work practitioners operate. They therefore need an understanding of the rationale and purposes of care management, and an understanding of how it will affect their work with people with dementia and their carers. This will help in deciding how to prioritise time, resources and energies. There is also an important obligation on social workers to identify and log needs that are not being met, and to challenge services creatively to begin to account for these.

In Chapter 3 we shall consider some of the skills, knowledge and values necessary for beginning social work practitioners, and relevant to experienced practitioners too.

3 Competence

Introduction

The centrality of competence in the practice of social work is emphasised in CCETSW's Paper 30, which details the requirements expected of social workers completing their education and training (CCETSW, 1995). The development of a competency-based approach to social work education is outlined by Yelloly (1995) and O'Hagan (1996). It stems from a desire to introduce clear standards and rigour into social work, and is dependent upon the assessment of clearly defined and observable criteria related to essential occupational tasks. In social work, the move to competency-based approaches began with the introduction of the Certificate of Social Service (CSS) in 1975 and has been advanced by the the introduction of the DipSW in 1989 and its revision in 1995. Jones (1995a) believes this trend has weakened the position of education and critical thinking in social work whilst giving emphasis to the voice of major state agencies. He considers competency-based training to be reductionist and to detract from questioning, thinking and developing creative responses to human need.

The charge of reductionism has been challenged. Competence can be seen as a broad concept which includes the need for flexibility and coping with unique and uncertain situations (Yelloly, 1995). There is also an emphasis on developing a secure knowledge base and working principles which allow the transfer of competence across situations.

Competences for practice are usually drawn from a comprehensive functional analysis of specific work-related tasks. The task is divided into small sub-units which comprise the larger whole. From these one can determine what it is one must do to achieve and demonstrate competence. In social work, a growing concern for practice competence in specific areas and a desire to address problems of recruitment from higher education led to the introduction of competency-based approaches in the DipSW.

Activity 3.1

What roles and functions are you likely to perform when working with people with dementia and their carers? What competences do you think you will need to do these well?

Comments

There are many different tasks and roles. These depend to a large extent on your work setting. They may include assessment, communication skills, management and organisation skills, planning and motivating. You may feel you need to have an in-depth knowledge of dementia or caregiving or communication and counselling techniques. You may also feel that you need guided experience in certain areas to increase your learning. Both the knowledge and experience will no doubt need a purpose and rationale, which may be found within the value base for social work which will be introduced later in this chapter.

The charges of reductionism have taken support from some individual models of behavioural thought which emphasise parts at the expense of the whole. However, as Jones and Joss (1995) point out, a more holistic approach can be taken which acknowledges that competences do not exist apart from wider contexts. The sub-tasks form part of a wider whole. In practice, competence in one area demands a knowledge of and practice within a set of circumstances which may differ from time to time. This perspective acknowledges that individuals bring their own values, culture and beliefs to their practice, and are themselves influenced by the setting and organisational culture in which they work. Whether we take a positive or negative view of competency-based social work, both perspectives agree that knowledge, skills and values develop within a context of practice experience. This is valued by proponents of both views (Jones, 1995a; Jones and Joss, 1995) and forms the basis of social work training as set out in the DipSW.

Two books concerning competence in social work practice and how it may be developed provide useful analyses and practice-based examples of this approach (O'Hagan, 1996; Vass, 1996). O'Hagan's work is interesting for its inclusion of a fairly comprehensive consideration of social work areas, but also because it does not include a chapter concerning social work competence in practice with older people. Mental health issues are included, and we may transfer the debate to working with people with dementia. Vass (1996) discusses competence in relation to community care practice and work with a range of adults in this context, but again, there is nothing specific to dementia.

Competence in social work

The term 'competence' is understood as the integration of knowledge, skills and values in practice situations.

Competence in working with people with dementia – which is the focus of this book – demands, among other knowledge, the acquisition of knowledge about dementia, the functioning of people with dementia, about carers, their location in wider social structures, the availability of resources and access to them. This is essential before one can provide effective intervention. But knowledge about what constitutes effective intervention is also necessary in developing competent social work practice. The skills to apply this knowledge and to recognise the impact of personal, client, carer, agency and cultural value systems are important to the purpose of social work.

CASE STUDY 3.1: PETER AND MARY

Peter Jones, a social work student with considerable prior experience in residential care, was asked to 'make an assessment of Mary Peters. She's got multi-infarct dementia and her daughter can't cope.' He was not sure what multi-infarct dementia was, what the daughter was supposed to cope with, and what in these circumstances constituted 'an assessment'.

In recognising these needs, he set about finding out what he could. He also sought time with the person making the request, and clarified matters with him.

Peter needed a range of knowledge about dementia, its effects, social and health service support and access to resources. He also needed the experience to learn to apply this knowledge but in a supervised and assisted way.

According to CCETSW (1995), the purpose of social work is:

> to enable children, adults, families, groups and communities to function, participate and develop in society. Social workers practise in a society of complexity, change and diversity, and the majority of people to whom they provide services, are among the most vulnerable and disadvantaged in that society. Social work-

ers are employed by a range of statutory, voluntary and private organizations, and work in collaboration with colleagues from allied professions and departments, as part of a network of welfare, health, housing, education and criminal justice provision. (p. 4)

In order to achieve this purpose, social workers must demonstrate their competence in the six core areas shown in Box 3.1.

Box 3.1   The six core competences for practice

1   Communicate and engage with organisations and people within communities to promote opportunities for children, adults, families and groups at risk or in need to function, participate and develop in society.
2   Promote opportunities for people to use their own strengths and expertise to enable them to meet responsibilities, secure rights and achieve change.
3   Work in partnership to assess and review people's circumstances and plan responses to need and risk.
4   Intervene and provide services to achieve change, through provision or purchase of appropriate levels of support, care, protection and control.
5   Contribute to the work of organisations.
6   Manage and evaluate your own capacity to develop professional competence.

The core competences are themselves broken down further into practice requirements, which provide smaller, but still fairly broad, tasks for completion to demonstrate competence. Paper 30 includes a range of evidence indicators for each practice requirement which demonstrate greater task-specific competence. When working with people with dementia it is important to show how completion of specific tasks meet the practice requirements in part fulfilment of the core competences.

What does this mean in practice? The social worker needs knowledge of:

- relevant legislation, including the Mental Health Act 1983, the National Health Service and Community Care Act 1990 and the Carers (Recognition and Services) Act 1995
- agency policy and procedure
- their personal role as a social worker

- the availability of a range of local resources
- family structure, dynamics, relationships, interactions and interconnections between patterns, scripts and present behaviours of the people they are working with
- a theoretical grounding in understanding families, caring, the impact of disease
- developmental needs of individuals, and an understanding of the processes of ageing and the impact of ageism at a personal, organisational and structural level
- optimal functioning, and barriers to optimal functioning in individuals
- models of mental health and dementia
- a variety of interventive techniques and their effectiveness
- recent research and its implications for practice.

Knowledge is gained by formal learning, application of understanding and experience, and reflection. It is not something static which can be imparted, but demands the full commitment of the learner. It is also important that knowledge is not seen in a vacuum apart from the context of skills needed to apply the knowledge and the values which underpin social work practice. Case study 3.2 will help you to consider the forms of knowledge necessary for competent practice, sources for this knowledge, and to begin to identify essential skills and values.

CASE STUDY 3.2: GEORGE AND MARGARET

George and Margaret Yavash had been married for forty years. They met in Cyprus, where Margaret's father was stationed in the army. After marrying, they came to England and settled to raise their family of three boys. The children had married, and the two eldest now had families of their own. They were a close family and visited regularly.

Margaret had been noticed to be increasingly forgetful over recent years. The family put this down to ageing. However, in the last six months the deterioration in her memory was more apparent. She had on numerous occasions burnt pans after forgetting they were on, had been brought back home by concerned individuals after forgetting why she had gone out, and had upset the whole family when she questioned who her son and grandchildren were, claiming that she did not know them.

George had relied upon Margaret to run the household while he had worked in his clothing business. He had now retired but still relied on Margaret for shopping, cleaning, cooking and making sure things ran smoothly. He felt that he could no longer cope with the situation and, at his request, his eldest son rang the social services for support and advice.

Activity 3.2

Many kinds of knowledge are necessary for effective and competent work in this case. It might help if you draw up a list of the sorts of knowledge you think is necessary.

Comments

Your list will no doubt include some of the following:

- a knowledge of the National Health Service and Community Care Act, to consider whether Margaret is entitled to an assessment and/or services
- the needs of the carers – perhaps especially George Yavash – are important, therefore an understanding of the implications of the Carers (Recognition and Services) Act is needed
- each local authority has different needs and services, so a knowledge of how local procedures and policies implement and operate this legislation is fundamental to applying the knowledge
- an understanding of family processes, patterns, scripts is important, to determine the impact of the present situation and needs arising from it
- also important in this regard is a knowledge of the importance and impact of cultural factors on family functioning
- a knowledge of dementia seems appropriate in this case; this may help in providing information, support, understanding and advice to the Yavashes and family
- knowledge of the impact of dementia on families and individuals, to help to plan effectively for present and future needs
- in order to intervene effectively, an up-to-date and comprehensive knowledge of what is available and how access can be gained to these resources
- a comprehensive knowledge of recent research, innovation and development in practice, to enable you to assist this family in the most effective way possible.

But knowledge on its own cannot deliver effective services. The social worker needs to be able to apply this knowledge. This demands a degree and level of skill which forms part of the competence for social work practice.

Skills must be put into practice. Prior learning and experiences are valuable resources to be drawn on, and to be enhanced and developed during education and training. In order to gain further skills in observation, assessment and practice, you should observe your own eco-system, family and friends, those of people you know, to develop knowledge of the vast range of optimal and good-enough living situations. This can also help in identifying and developing listening and communication skills.

A number of social work skills are necessary to apply the knowledge effectively and competently in the case of Margaret Yavash. These include:

- assessment skills
- interviewing skills
- interpersonal skills
- communication skills with people with dementia
- co-ordination and management skills
- report-writing skills
- skills in negotiation and liaison with other agencies/professionals.

The majority of these skills can be subsumed under the broad heading 'communication or interpersonal skills', but it is worth separating them out because they each refer to a different aspect of the case study.

In order to understand the situation and needs of each person involved in the situation, the social worker must be competent in making assessments. This will involve knowledge of dementia, the impact of family and social factors, knowledge of resources, policies, procedures and legislation. In making assessments, however, the social worker will need to plan a range of visits and interviews, will need to demonstrate good listening and interpersonal skills, be able to put people at their ease and collect relevant information. The social worker must also be able to record this information accurately, be able to communicate, negotiate and liaise with other agencies who can supply services to meet identified needs, and to co-ordinate and manage the process. Importantly, the social worker will need to develop skills in monitoring and reviewing the effectiveness of the process.

Activity 3.3

What skills do you think you might need to plan adequately for Case study 3.2?

Comment

You will no doubt have identified assessment and communication skills. These are key components of effective practice. The Yavash family have a number of needs resulting from changing roles and circumstances. As a social worker, it will be your job to assess these needs for safe skills within the home, adequate completion and what, if any, services are needed, and from where these may be obtained. This will entail talking with Margaret and George and others involved, seeking wants and wishes, matching these against potential risks, and acquiring services if necessary.

Knowledge and values are important to the effective delivery of social work services. They are complemented and underpinned by values. It is important to know why social work is practised and what system of values underpins it. In this way the skills become less technical and more human, and the knowledge becomes focused on the concerns of a holistic approach to the person.

The values element of competence is emphasised in social work. At present six values are highlighted:

1   Identify and question your own values and prejudices, and their implications for practice.
2   Respect and value uniqueness and diversity, and recognise and build on strengths.
3   Promote people's rights to choice, privacy, confidentiality and protection, while recognising and addressing the complexities of competing rights and demands.
4   Assist people to increase control of and improve the quality of their lives, while recognising that control of behaviour will be required at times in order to protect children and adults from harm.
5   Identify, analyse and take action to counter discrimination, racism, disadvantage, inequality and injustice, using strategies appropriate to role and context.
6   Practise in a manner that does not stigmatise or disadvantage either individuals, groups or communities.

Box 3.2 Values and social work with older people

- a commitment to equality of access to services and the basic rights of citizenship

- a respect for independence and self-determination, minimising restraint and allowing risk-taking

- a regard for privacy, minimising intrusion, providing confidentiality

- an understanding of the individuality and dignity of every service user and carer

- a quest to maximise individual choice in services

- provision of services to promote realisation of an individual's aspirations and abilities in all aspects of daily life

- acknowledgement of the value older people have for society

- the right to take informed risks and acknowledgement that the quality of an older person's life is paramount

- the right to privacy

- the right to dignity, acknowledgement of the role of informal carers

- the right to chocie

- the right to independence and fulfilment regardless of race, sex, disability or cultural background

Sources: SSI (1991, para 81) Winner (1992).

Whilst these are broad and cover all aspects of social work practice, they encompass the values outlined by the Social Services Inspectorate (1991) and CCETSW's concern for good practice with older people (Winner, 1992 – see Box 3.2).

The social worker for Margaret Yavash and family needs to be aware of their own value base, fears and thoughts of ageing and illness in order to practise without hidden agendas influencing the course of the work. It is important in this case to be aware of the potential impact of cultural factors on the family functioning, the ways in which matters are dealt with, and the impact of the dementia and deterioration in functioning seen. It is also important to recognise that cultural stereotypes must not be imposed on the basis of different ethnic origins. Each person or family worked with should be seen as unique, and the response and needs also as unique. Thus values of anti-oppressive practice need to be at the forefront of social work practice to be effective and competent.

It will be important for the social worker to find out the wants, wishes and needs of all involved, and to work towards some way of addressing these which maintains privacy, dignity, choice and independence and also protects from harm and danger. The social worker must employ the skills of diplomacy and negotiation in dealing with potentially conflicting needs and wants, and allow the voice of all to be heard. Margaret Yavash must be allowed her chance to determine her needs, and George Yavash also has needs as a carer which will influence care planning.

Summary

Determining needs and applying social work values demands a high level of skill, increased by experience and by the utilisation of a clear framework of knowledge for practice. The integration of knowledge, skills and values is essential for competent social work practice in all fields. The complexities of working with people with dementia and their families demands such competence and effectiveness. Knowledge, skills and values underpin many of the approaches which have developed in social work and the helping professions.

In Part II of this book we will introduce a comprehensive range of strategies for effective and competent work with people with dementia and their families. These can be used in all areas of practice, from day care, residential care to field work and community work.

Part II

Models for practice

There are few social work texts concerning dementia care which provide detailed practice guidance on many methods. There are, of course, many excellent texts about aspects of dementia care, and these have been referred to in the earlier chapters. In this part we offer an overview of a range of methods to help the practitioner ensure that practice is appropriate, positive and enhances the values of dignity, respect and personhood of people with dementia and their carers. People do not live in isolation, and the wider perspective, including carers and significant others, will be referred to throughout this section.

The methods are wide-ranging and are underpinned by different theoretical positions and knowledge. These are not necessarily mutually exclusive. Although it is quite right to guard against eclecticism and to understand the models and approaches employed, an approach using different models with the same people but in different circumstances can be refreshing, validating and demonstrate commitment to those involved and their needs.

The part will begin with an examination of crisis intervention, since many of those with whom social work practitioners come into contact do so at a point of crisis. This will be followed by a consideration of action-oriented and behavioural methods, psychotherapeutic and person-focused methods, and finally by a brief excursus into the use of community and empowerment/advocacy work.

4 Crisis intervention

Introduction

Most people only come into contact with social services at a point of crisis. The stigma of the workhouse and the Poor Law still remains, and may be one reason why this is the case. Another reason may be the increased emphasis on self-reliance promoted throughout the 1980s. This chapter will examine crisis, its meaning and potential uses for people with dementia and their carers.

CASE STUDY 4.1: NORMAN AND ELLIE

Norman Scott-Brown was 76. He lived with his second wife, Ellie, in a large flat on the outskirts of the city. During World War II he had served in Burma and had spent two years as a prisoner of war. Since returning to England after the war he had suffered from recurring nightmares and cycles of anxiety and depression. Ellie described how these episodes had led to the break-up of his first marriage. Ellie said she knew about his 'nerves' before marrying him, and could understand why he sometimes felt like this. However, she had become increasingly concerned about him over recent months.

Norman was said to be forgetting things more frequently, although his memory had never been very good. He even mixed up Ellie and his first wife, which, she said, hurt her considerably. Ellie realised that something must be wrong when Norman missed his monthly meeting of the Burma Star Society and became verbally and physically aggressive towards her when she mentioned it. She said it was as though he knew he should remember something, but being reminded of it simply reinforced the idea

51

that something was amiss. Over the following few months further changes occurred. He began retreating into past times, especially the days in which he was a prisoner of war. This was very distressing for both Norman and Ellie. He seemed to lose his bearings around the flat, although they had lived there for fifteen years. The final straw came when he forgot the names of his son and family when they came to visit. He became very angry and shouted at Ellie blaming her for poisoning him.

Ellie rang social services for some assistance in dealing with these changes. She was adamant that she wished to continue looking after him and providing him with the care he needed, but she did not know if she could cope with the uncertainty and changes in his memory and temperament. The doctor thought Norman was suffering from Alzheimer's disease and requested an assessment from the local day hospital. This preliminary diagnosis worried Ellie. She was afraid of the extra demands it might put her under, and believed she might not cope with the situation.

A few weeks after the initial involvement of social services a call was received from the police, who had found Norman in the street at three o'clock in the morning. He told the police he was getting out before he too was killed. After calming him down they returned him home, but felt that he was in need of extra care and support. The social worker who visited found him very confused and liable to swing in his mood. She also thought that Ellie was under considerable strain. The social worker was unsure whether to seek an approved social work assessment or not.

The model and approach

Before we can discuss crisis intervention work and assess its uses and limitations when working with people with dementia and their carers, we need to examine how the term 'crisis' is used and what it means. Having done this, we will be in a position to discuss crisis intervention and to review some of its applications within social work.

What is a crisis?

We all have some ideas of what it is that constitutes a crisis. These may include personal crises such as failing an exam or a relationship ending, or more objective crises such as a natural disaster. In the helping professions, however, the word has assumed a more technical meaning.

One of the pioneers of crisis intervention described a crisis as:

> a time-limited period of psychological disequilibrium, precipitated by a sudden significant change in a person's life situation, which results in demands for

internal adaptation and external adjustment which for the time being are not possible for the individual to achieve. (Caplan, 1961, p. 41)

This understanding has endured (Roberts, 1991). A crisis reflects individuals' responses to a situation with which they cannot deal using their existing ways of coping. Crises demand new ways of acting, but they are time-limited.

There are two basic types of crisis:

1 *accidental or situational crises* – these reflect reactions to unexpected traumatic events, for instance when a previously healthy person has a stroke and loses mental and physical abilities.
2 *developmental crises* – reactions to life transitions or maturational stages, such as retirement, which, if not planned for, may constitute a crisis for those involved.

A crisis, therefore, differs from an emergency (Getz et al., 1974), although many people may confuse the two. The impact on individuals and their perceptions constitutes the crisis, rather than the event itself (O'Hagan, 1986; Miller, 1963; Bloom, 1963). When particular events are associated with crises, such as bereavement, ill health or loss of employment, this may single out people experiencing distress in other situations for blame or dismissal of the seriousness of their experiences. People generally learn to discriminate between situations and actions, and behave according to the values of their culture and society. However, if their capacity for mental reasoning and grasp of social situations is impaired, their reactions may also be unexpected. For people with dementia it may be increasingly difficult to live and act within the expected rules of society. This may exacerbate their distress and, as mentioned in Chapter 1 attract negative comments and treatment from others.

It is also important to acknowledge cultural diversity in response to certain events and triggers. Past experiences of our culture, society and families create a range of different individual responses. Such an understanding of crisis allows us to see individuals as unique, and not to apportion blame according to their reactions to events and failure to cope in certain situations.

Whatever the event or situation precipitating the crisis, it seems that there are certain key features involved in the experience of crises. Parry (1990) suggests that these comprise:

- a precipitating event or the result of long-term stress
- individually experienced distress
- a sense of loss, danger to the self or humiliation
- feelings of being out of control of the situation

- unexpected events
- disruption of usual patterns and routines
- uncertainty about the future
- the distress continues over time, although this is limited.

Not all is bleak, however, as a crisis represents a turning point – a time of *danger* and *opportunity* – the danger of being overwhelmed, and the opportunity of learning more adaptive coping mechanisms and accepting help from others (Aguilera and Messick, 1974, 1982). A crisis is self-limiting, and resolution – for better or for worse – occurs soon after onset. This presents a time of opportunity for constructive change (Caplan, 1961).

People's desire to lessen their distress increases their willingness to change. Crisis intervention is effective at this time (Baldwin, 1979; Aguilera and Messick, 1982; Olsen, 1984; Golan, 1978). If they resolve the crisis well, it is likely that they will deal adaptively with future hazardous events and situations. The converse is also true. Successful resolution may be defined in individual ways. It is important to seek the views of those with whom you are working, to establish what it is that constitutes success and to work towards this goal.

Crises do not only occur for individuals but happen in families and groups. One benefit of seeing the crisis in a systemic way is that attention and blame is deflected from one individual out towards all members of the family and wider systems affected by the crisis situation (O'Hagan, 1986). This may be particularly important when working with people with dementia. The crisis may not only affect them but may also affect carers and others in contact with that person. It also allows each situation to be seen as unique. A summary of these ideas is given in Box 4.1.

Box 4.1   The characteristics of crises

- Crises are emotionally distressing situations in which a person's usual coping methods do not work and the individual feels out of control
- Individual perceptions are fundamental, but others are involved and crises can be understood systemically
- Individual weakness or blame is not conferred by this understanding of a crisis. Social and cultural factors are important
- Crises are time-limited
- Resolution can be for good or ill
- Motivation for change is enhanced during a crisis.

Activity 4.1

Make a list of some types of crisis and the principal components of a crisis. Use your understanding of dementia care to suggest situations in which these apply.

Comment

Crisis situations are, as we have seen, potentially unlimited. However, there are two basic types: those which happen without prior warning, and those which we can foresee to some extent. What characterises the experience is the perception that an individual cannot cope with a situation or event, and that the person's usual ways of dealing with such situations do not seem to work.

In dementia care you may have noted the experience of receiving an initial diagnosis. Whilst the fact that something was amiss may be foreseen, it is not something that can be planned for. It may lead to despondency and feelings of being overwhelmed by the person and by his or her carer. Both may feel unable to cope with the demands and losses associated with the diagnosis. It is at this stage that social work support is necessary, however. Crisis points hold both dangers and opportunities, and people are more open to developing new skills and coping strategies to deal with their distress. If the opportunity is missed, however, it may be that the person with dementia and the carers simply develop ways of lessening the emotional distress without working through associated issues and problems. The crisis may pass, but coping skills may be diminished.

Historical and theoretical development

Crisis theory and crisis intervention have a long history of development. Roberts (1991) refers to Hippocrates's understanding of the importance of crises in medicine and health as far back as 400 BC.

The conceptual and theoretical origins are varied. The theoretical base has developed in sophistication from its psychoanalytic beginnings, especially following Lindemann's (1944) study of grief reactions after a nightclub fire in Coconut Grove, Boston. Crisis theory has also developed from:

- developmental psychology (Erikson, 1950; Parkes, 1971)
- ego psychology (Hartmann, 1958)
- person-centred approaches (Rogers, 1951; Getz et al., 1974)

- gestalt therapy (Perls et al., 1973)
- systems thinking (Langsley, 1968; Aguilera and Messick, 1982; O'Hagan, 1986)
- stress theory and social learning theory (Rapoport, 1970; Thompson, 1991; Dattilio and Freeman, 1994).

This varied theoretical background has led to a wide-ranging adoption of the concepts and usefulness of crisis theory by practitioners from a range of disciplines, with different styles and approaches and working with different client groups.

Models of crisis development

Many different models have developed, but perhaps the American psychiatrist Gerald Caplan is the best-known name associated with crisis intervention. His work has been instrumental in the development of the concept and its application to mental health. He saw four stages in the development of the crisis (see Box 4.2).

Box 4.2 Caplan's model of crisis

1 an initial rise in tension caused by the problem stimulus.
2 an increase in tension because the problem remains unresolved.
3 a further increase in tension, compelling the individual to attempt new methods of resolution, redefining and compartmentalising the problem.
4 if problem remains unresolved, tension may mount beyond an individual's threshold, leading to a major disorganisation of that individual, with dramatic results.

Baldwin (1981) provides a comprehensive description of the phases involved in an emotional crisis. Like Caplan, he proposes four stages, but the latter two are separated into adaptive and maladaptive resolution sections (see Box 4.3).

From these understandings and conceptualisations a number of interventive models have developed. Figure 4.1 provides a diagram of crisis theory and intervention which may be applied to practice situations.

Box 4.3 Baldwin's crisis model (Baldwin 1981)

Phase one: The emotionally hazardous situation

a An increase in uncomfortable feelings signals disruption of homoeostatic balance.

b Discomfort motivates attempts to reduce it.

c Usual coping mechanisms are employed.

d Usual coping behaviours are, in most cases, successful in returning the individual to homoeostasis in a short period of time.

Phase two: The emotional crisis

a Usual coping strategies are ineffective.

b Discomfort intensifies and thought distortions increase.

c Novel coping behaviours and problem-solving techniques are employed to reduce the crisis.

d The individual seeks help and support from others.

Phase three: Crisis resolution

Adaptive resolution

a Help allows the individual to deal successfully with affective and cognitive issues and learn new problem-solving and coping behaviours.

b Underlying conflicts raised by the crisis are identified. Work to resolve them is put into action.

c Internal and external sources of help and support are put into operation.

d Affective disquiet is reduced and there is a return to *at least* the pre-crisis level of functioning.

Maladaptive resolution

a Novel problem-solving and coping strategies are not learned and adequate help is not sought or found.

b Underlying conflicts remain unresolved.

c Internal and external sources of help and support are not operationalised.

d Affective disquiet is reduced but the individual functions at a less adaptive level.

Phase four: Post-crisis adaptation

Adaptive resolution

a The individual becomes less vulnerable in similar situations because of problem and past conflict resolution.

b Novel and adaptive coping skills and problem-solving behaviours have been learned.

c Individual functioning may have improved and personal growth may have taken place.

d The likelihood of similar future emotionally hazardous situations developing into a crisis is reduced.

Maladaptive resolution

a The individual is more vulnerable than before because of a failure to deal effectively with underlying conflicts.

b The individual has learned maladaptive strategies to cope with emotionally hazardous situations.

c General functioning may be less adaptive than before the crisis.

d Future similar emotionally hazardous situations may be more likely to develop into crises.

Source: Baldwin (1981).

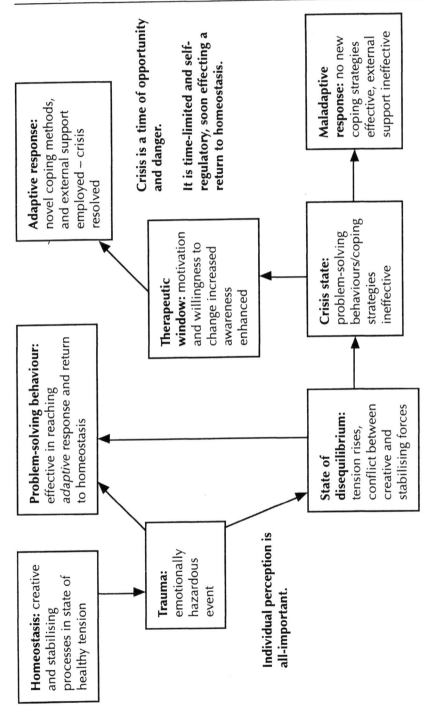

Figure 4.1   The crisis process

The many applications of crisis theory

Crisis intervention has been used with positive results in many settings with many different client groups, including:

- suicide (McGee, 1974; Newhill, 1993; Hoff, 1989)
- mental health issues (Caplan, 1961, 1964; Parad, 1965; Langsley, 1968; Echlin and Ramon, 1992; Tamayo et al., 1990) and physical ill health (Woolley, 1990; Christ et al., 1991)
- domestic violence (Hoff, 1990)
- rape crisis (Scott, 1993; Edlis, 1993)
- children and families (Lapernieve, 1993; Webb, 1991; Stevenson and Grauerholz, 1993)
- national or major disaster (Hayes et al., 1990; Hodgkinson and Stewart, 1991; Toft and Reynolds, 1994).

Practice models for crisis intervention

There are many different models for the practical application of crisis intervention. We will focus on problem-solving models that accord well with behavioural and task-focused work but also employ the skills of counselling.

Aguilera (1990) lists a number of steps involved in her problem-solving approach to crisis intervention. Following from a comprehensive assessment and a period of planning, the intervention itself is implemented. She states that this is highly dependent upon the client's pre-existing skills, and the creativity and flexibility of the practitioner. However, four particular steps are considered integral to the model:

1 *Helping the client to understand their crisis in an intellectual way* – thus the practitioner can describe the relationship between the crisis and the trigger or precipitating event.
2 *Helping the client to vent feelings* – this may involve the expression of feelings hitherto suppressed in some way.
3 *Exploration of coping mechanisms* – this includes an examination of alternative and existing methods of coping.
4 *Re-opening the social world* – this is particularly important where there has been significant loss.

The problem-solving approach involves a sequence of logical reasoning, although not always a set of well-defined steps. It may involve 'reproductive problem-solving' which depends to a large extent upon past successes in dealing with crisis situations, or if no such experiences are available, 'productive problem-solving'. This employs resources hitherto unused – novel – ways of coping. The individual must construct new ideas and solutions, for which she proposes a five-stage interventive plan (see Box 4.4).

Box 4.4   A five-stage crisis intervention plan

1   **Assessment of the individual and the problem**: What was the trigger, and what factors continue to interfere with the individual's ability to solve problems? The focus should be upon the immediate problem, not an in-depth exploration of the individual's past history. Usual coping skills, available supports, and individual meaning represent important considerations at this stage.

2   **The planning of therapeutic intervention**: An assessment of the impact on the individual's life and those around him or her is necessary. Thinking through this may lead to a consideration of alternatives and an evaluation of these in the context of past experiences and knowledge as well as the needs of the present. An understanding of why the problem exists and tentative causal relationships may appear.

3   **Intervention**: After the problem is identified, alternative solutions can be explored in order to reduce the symptoms of stress and anxiety. The alternatives should be evaluated as objectively as possible in terms of the individual's functioning.

4   **Resolution of the crisis**: The subjective meaning of the crisis plays an important role in determining the nature and degree of coping behaviours. Realistic perception allows the individual to see the relationship between the event and feelings of stress, and is necessary to effective resolution.

5   **Anticipatory planning**: Available situational supports need to be identified and employed to ensure future adaptive functioning. Lifestyle and learned coping mechanisms should be identified and practised in anticipation of new, potentially stressful situations.

Objections may be voiced immediately to the use of such an approach with a person with short-term memory problems. For instance, how able are they to develop productive strategies for resolving the crisis, and can they understand the link between events and perceptions? It is here that we find the use of eco-systems – the wider network in which the person lives and interacts – to be important. Crises do not occur in isolation from other factors which have an impact on people's lives. Changes in one part of the wider system influence other parts, including the person with failing cognitive abilities.

Burgess and Baldwin (1981) have taken the two divergent models of screening and assessment (derived from psychoanalytic principles) and problem-solving (derived from person-centred and action-oriented traditions) and conflated them. Their 'convergence model' has a past–present–future orientation. This allows individuals in crisis to work through reactivated past conflicts while focusing on the present situation, and has as its goal the return to at least a pre-crisis level of functioning, or even the enhancement of future coping.

Whichever particular model is chosen, practitioners must have at their disposal a number of qualities and skills. The ability to create and maintain an effective time-goal contract is a major determinant of the outcome of intervention (Burgess and Baldwin, 1981). This is also important when working with people with dementia and their families. It assists in promoting clarity, maintaining a focus and in concentrating on agreed problems between all parties. Of course, the capacity of the individual to make agreements may be reduced, and there is a danger of agreements being made which do not reflect the wishes and needs of the individual. It is the social worker's role here to ensure that each party has a voice, that all issues are raised and that collusion is minimised. By developing an agreement which is overseen by individual, family and carers, social worker and his or her supervisor, some of these dangers can be reduced.

Crises, as we have seen, are time-limited, and people are at their most susceptible to change and external influence during a crisis. The crisis intervention practitioner needs a certain emotional maturity to deal constructively with reality, must be able to adapt to change, must be relatively free of anxieties, needs the capacity to find satisfaction in giving, and must relate to others consistently (Getz et al., 1974). Interpersonal skills are essential. The practitioner must be able to communicate in verbal and non-verbal ways. He or she must use communication to direct the client towards goal accomplishment, to facilitate expression, to analyse interpersonal processes, and to evaluate and work at the pace of the client.

The crisis intervention practitioner must also develop a self-awareness and understanding of his or her emotions, and how he or she has functioned in crisis situations. This aids the expression of the three core skills of genuineness, empathy and warmth.

Burgess and Baldwin (1981) describe three levels of skills necessary to the crisis intervention practitioner (see Box 4.5).

Box 4.5   Crisis intervention skills

- **Conceptual skills** – for understanding client problems and developing strategies for change
- **Clinical skills** – this extends the conceptual framework to implementing effective intervention
- **Communication skills** – for information exchange.

Activity 4.2

Think of the models for crisis intervention reviewed above. Which do you think would be applicable to your work with people with dementia? Why do you think this?

Comment

You may feel that problem-solving models have potential but are fraught with difficulties because of the mental skills and judgements needed. However, you may see potential in individual cases, depending on the social supports a person has and that person's individual reaction to the dementia.

If we take the example of the reaction to the initial diagnosis considered in Case study 4.1, we may be able to suggest possibilities for using a problem-solving model. The initial assessment would focus on existing coping skills and supports. It may be that the person has acted as the main emotional and practical support for a partner or relative, and possible changes in roles and expectations would need to be explored. It may be that alternative options and future planning would be required to ensure that roles and tasks were continued in the person's preferred way, with the support from other sources being commissioned if so required and requested. The main focus of the work might legitimately focus on the perceptions of those involved, and whilst confronting the situation, emphasising the existing skills a person has and that continued abilities are indeed possible.

Having reviewed crisis theory and a number of practice models, we must turn now to a consideration of how crisis intervention may be used in Case study 4.1.

CASE STUDY 4.2: NORMAN AND ELLIE

Initially, the social worker needed to assess the situation and account for any immediate needs and concerns. She was worried that the situation was out of hand and specialist advice might be necessary. To this end she arranged for an approved social work assessment, which determined that it would be more beneficial to keep Norman at home if possible. A first task for the social worker, therefore, was to determine whether or not there was a crisis, and for whom.

Ellie had reached the end of her coping capacity. She was trying new ways of dealing with the situation by mobilising outside supports, which certainly demonstrated a positive strength but did not at that time reduce the problems she was experiencing.

It was more difficult for Norman. Throughout his life he had experienced emotional disquiet and feelings of being out of control. Usually these were dealt with over time with the assistance of his doctor. This was not the case in this instance, and his frustration was leading to displays of temper and violent outbursts. Since his memory problems had become more noticeable and his frustration more pronounced, tension had risen, and this was not reduced by Ellie's support. The worker involved was led to believe that the changes in his memory and functioning and the perceptions Ellie had of the diagnosis constituted a crisis for both of them.

It was important that the social worker dealt honestly and openly with the diagnosis and changes in memory, functioning and social activities which appeared to constitute the main trigger events. By providing time and allowing Norman and Ellie to vent their feelings and, at times, to rage against the situation, it was possible to defuse a crisis that was likely to become an emergency necessitating greater amounts of care and possibly separating them. Talking through the situation and their feelings allowed them to offload, to reduce tension and to work out their wants and wishes for future care.

In negotiation with Ellie and paying attention to her wants and wishes, the social worker made an agreement to provide support and advice to her on a regular basis. At the time, Ellie did not wish to receive practical support such as home help, day care or respite care, but said that she needed to know that these were available and attainable should she change her mind at a later date. She did, however, want to attend the local carers' support group. This agreement provided a contact in case future needs arose, helped to begin to provide further education and information via the support group, and opened up new avenues of social contact and support for Ellie.

The social worker emphasised the strengths of the couple. Ellie had developed a clear understanding of Norman's emotional and psychological needs over the years, together they had worked out plans for support when things became difficult, they were prepared to use outside supports and they had a strong relationship. These strengths were built upon by the provision of information and support.

Education concerning possible future changes and expectations helped them to plan future solutions to potential difficulties. They both appreciated having a degree of control and the social worker co-ordinating but not leading. Ellie and Norman began to talk more when planning future care and anticipating future needs. This lowered the tension that had arisen between them, and gave them the chance to re-establish their relationship in the light of changed circumstances.

The provision of education and information reduced some of the impact of the negative perceptions arising from Ellie's understanding of dementia, and assisted her in relocating her concerns in the context of a caring and enduring relationship. Having said this, it was done in the context of openness and full knowledge of potential future difficulties.

The social work role was one of co-ordination, locating resources and supports, providing a vent to feelings and anger, and providing information and education. The overall function was case manager, and she had the responsibility to review changing and future needs as they arose. It is difficult to say what might have happened if work had not proceeded in this way, but it is likely that resolution of the crisis would have been maladaptive, resulting in a failure to cope, a breakdown in care and an increase in tension and potential violence. This timely intervention was cost-effective in reducing the need for expensive support such as residential care and dealing with greater trauma and upset.

Crisis intervention and social work with people with dementia and their carers

Social work with people with dementia presents a unique challenge. Progressive or incremental cognitive decline and difficulties in learning new material or living skills make any intervention, especially problem-solving, particularly difficult. However, during the early stages of the disease it may still be possible to learn new ways of adapting and coping. This may be especially important when the diagnosis is first made, which may be the trigger for a potential crisis. The stress involved in caring for someone deteriorating in personality, cognition and general functioning, and increased fear of the disease process, are understandably significant and emotionally hazardous events that may precipitate crises where outside help is needed to regain a former level of functioning. It must be remembered that individual humans are generally part of larger living systems, and changes effected within the people they live with or are close to or significant to them in some way may resolve a crisis situation. It is important to decide who is in crisis.

Most referrals in which dementia is an issue are made at points of crisis, although of course not all. For a variety of reasons, including pride, embarrassment and fear exacerbated by the media, people often do not contact social services unless there appears to be no alternative. In making a referral, it can be noted that the referring agent often presents a solution rather than a request, and this is often, as O'Hagan (1986) notes, *a plea for removal*. This places a heavy burden upon social workers. The initial assessment and intervention – including the provision of practical help, support and reassurance, advice and further referral when appropriate – can, as seen in the context of crisis theory, influence the outcome of that situation for good or ill. All social work skills must be employed towards effecting a constructive resolution of the crisis, such as advocacy, bargaining, negotiation, challenging and empathy, and the individual's preferred method of intervention. The legal context of the National Health Service and Community Care Act 1990 demands choice, flexibility and an enabling approach. Crisis intervention offers just such a framework, and there is certainly ample evidence of its effectiveness, as mentioned earlier.

A primary worker task is to determine whose the crisis is, and then to attempt to resolve that situation by adaptive means, perhaps using one of the models introduced above. The intervention must take into account all participants in a living system, not simply the person in crisis, and must manipulate that system – in an ethical manner – to a position in which they are enabled to function as adaptively and constructively as possible. A model for use is presented in Figure 4.2.

A crisis may also develop for professionals involved in a case. The end result may again be adaptive or maladaptive, and the need for supervisors and managers to utilise the individual crisis situation for workers is self-evident. An example of a maladaptive response would be to use the Mental Health Act 1983 or section 47 of the National Assistance Act 1948 to effect removal to residential care or hospital, or in some circumstances not to act, because of insufficient resources, panic in the practitioner, or a practitioner acting in collusion with a psychiatrist, police officer, relative or neighbour rather than advocating on behalf of the person with dementia and protecting their rights.

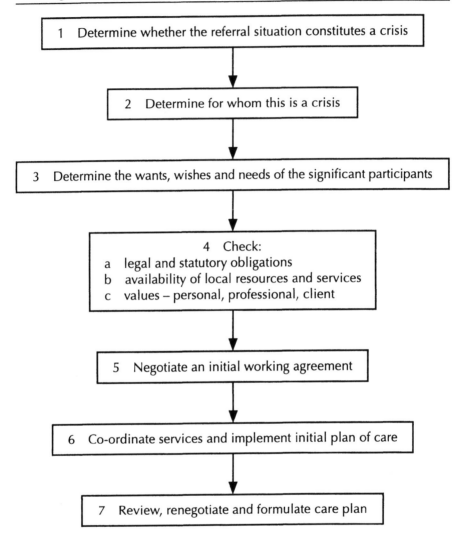

Figure 4.2   Crisis intervention flowchart

A specific objection to crisis intervention is raised where dementia is an issue: that crisis intervention is not viable for people with dementia because of their cognitive deficits and impaired potential for learning.

Among the first noticeable symptoms of Alzheimer's disease and some of the other diseases causing dementia, problems in learning and memory are common, but the assessment of learning deficits is difficult (Raaijmakers and Abbenhuis, 1992) because of the uniqueness of manifestation in each person.

It must also be remembered that in early dementia many people retain some capacity for new learning, and a high level of awareness of their failures of competence and life changes (Froggatt, 1988). We have also noted that crises occur within living systems, and adaptation involving other parts of this system, for example family members or carers, may change perceptions of crisis situations even when an individual no longer has the capacity for volitional adaptation. Personal attention to the individual with dementia has positive ramifications for their sense of wellbeing (Kitwood, 1990; Feil, 1992, 1993).

There are other objections and misconceptions, and it is to these that we must now turn.

It is hoped that the preceding discussion has laid most of these to rest. Burgess and Baldwin (1981) discuss a number of misconceptions. The main ones are repeated here.

- *Crisis intervention is only valuable for responding to psychiatric emergencies.* This, as we have seen, derives in part from the misconception that a crisis is synonymous with an emergency, and the literature reviewed demonstrates its wide-ranging effectiveness
- *Crisis intervention is a 'one-shot' form of therapy.* Although some clients do only need one visit it is more often the case that intervention ranges from one to eight sessions in quite an intensive but time-limited period
- *Crisis intervention is practised by paraprofessionals.* This criticism developed in the USA, and referred mainly to the problem-solving techniques that developed in drug and substance abuse agencies in the 1960s. In fact, crisis intervention has been practised by a wide range of professionals with a variety of different client groups
- *Crisis intervention does not produce lasting change.* The potential for adaptive change and the enhancement of future coping is clear in crisis intervention literature.

To these misconceptions we must add the following (see Parker, 1992):

- *Crisis Intervention comes too late. Prevention is better than cure.* Most referrals to social workers are made at times of crisis, and not at a time when preventive action might have been possible. Should an adaptive response be the outcome following crisis intervention, the potential for coping may well be increased, or at least brought back to the level before the crisis
- *Crisis intervention is merely an excuse for a lack of resources, and it would not be used if there were adequate resources.* Even if adequate resources were allocated to the personal social services, referrals would still be

made at times of crisis. The intention of crisis intervention is to be enabling, to effect change, and not to be disabling. Crisis intervention is not crisis management and not second best, but a constructive beginning framework for social work intervention

- *There is a danger that all referrals may be seen as crises and responded to in this way, and consequently intervention would be ineffective.* It is necessary to determine whether the situation constitutes a crisis, and a full grounding in crisis theory and its application in practice is evidently needed in order to ensure effectiveness and appropriateness of intervention

- *There are ethical problems with crisis intervention. Self-determination is not possible, and the worker seeks to manipulate the situation, thus leading to many possible abuses and unethical decisions.* This is, of course, possible, but the ethical underpinning of the social work role committed to anti-discriminatory practice and open participation should guard against such possibilities. Also, the statutory framework in which crisis intervention is to be practised is enabling, creating choice, and empowering in terms of future coping. In fact, given the potential for constructive change that intervening in a crisis situation allows, failing to employ crisis intervention may itself be unethical, since contingencies may not be manipulated that would avoid a potentially damaging and painful crisis when the lack of change demonstrated by usual coping strategies becomes evident because of a rise in tension levels. In this case, enabling a service user to employ a novel coping strategy may offset not only a crisis but also a permanent deterioration in functioning

- *Crisis intervention is judgemental.* The use of crisis theory is often linked to approaches where 'something' is said to be wrong and in need of fixing (Howe, 1987). Given that our definition of 'crisis' places it not only in its environmental and systemic context but also in terms of relativity and subjectivity, this view may need some modification.

Activity 4.3

What do you see as the main benefits and limitations of using crisis intervention in your work with people with dementia and their carers?

Comment

You may perhaps not feel that the objections or the possibilities listed in this chapter are applicable to your work. Perhaps you work in continuing care, day or residential care, and feel that people simply need consistent and frequent care services matched to their individual needs and according to agreed care plans. This is important. However, people receiving continuing input, high levels of services and support are still prone to crisis situations. A carer's sudden admission to hospital, a bereavement, increased confusion and forgetfulness or the loss of a skill can all precipitate a crisis. It is important to realise when this occurs in order to maximise the potential for a good resolution for all concerned.

A major benefit but also a potential limitation in crisis intervention is the power to manipulate the situation and people's coping abilities for good or ill. It is essential for social workers to keep clearly in focus the value base which protects and champions the rights and responsibilities of individuals. A small intervention may effect considerable change. Rather than simply reacting and perhaps seeking a residential placement for someone whose carer cannot continue because of ill health or hospitalisation, for instance, it is important to assess functioning, activities of daily living, other supports and the wants and wishes of those involved. Crisis intervention may provide a creative and respectful approach to crisis situations.

Summary

Many referrals are made in crisis situations, and it is unlikely that this will change even with the allocation of greater resources to social services departments. The development of the crisis is not observed in these situations, so preventive action is often not possible. However, in existing situations an understanding of the developmental process leading to crisis will be influential in undertaking preventive work.

Crisis intervention provides a unique opportunity to effect constructive change, to intervene in order to optimise social functioning, to enable choice and participation, and to provide appropriate services. Given the possibilities for change, intervening in crises offers the practitioner a chance to build trust, rapport and work in partnership with service users to honour the values common to social work and the new legislation – that individual choice should be respected and maximised, and that people should be enabled rather than disabled and objectified.

Because it is a crisis that often brings people with dementia and their carers into contact with social workers, this chapter has preceded other ways of working. There is, however, a clear link to action-oriented approaches, and it is to these that we shall now turn.

5 Cognitive-behavioural approaches

Introduction

Whatever we *do* may be classed as behaviour, but it is also much more than this. Whilst behaviour is the observable action of people acting in response to, within, on and as part of their wider social environment, it is also the product of our thoughts and deliberations about how we ought to act in particular situations and under particular circumstances. Behaviour has a thinking or *cognitive* element to it.

Cognitive-behavioural work refers to the systematic alteration of behaviour by increasing, decreasing or maintaining it. It involves altering the triggers to and consequences of behaviours. The main aim is to increase pro-social behaviours and to reduce the expression of anti-social or unhelpful behaviours.

Unfortunately, however, cognitive-behavioural work has had a 'bad press' since it has been associated with some of the more 'aversive' and punishment-based techniques, whilst little attention has been paid to the constructive and adaptive elements of behavioural practice (Sheldon, 1995; Parker and Randall, 1997b).

The approach seeks to understand human behaviour in its social context. A basic presupposition is that if behaviour is learnt then it can be unlearnt, or new behaviours can be learnt to replace less useful ones. It is the concern of people using these approaches to widen the range of possible responses that an individual can make to their environment, and to be able to change it, and not to limit, direct and determine people's actions. In this sense it is a highly ethical approach that accords with the codes of ethics of social care professional bodies (BASW, 1975; CCETSW, 1995).

Whilst there are many theories of learning, we shall concentrate on four:

1   respondent or classical conditioning.
2   operant or instrumental conditioning.
3   modelling, imitative or vicarious learning.
4   cognitive-behavioural theories.

Each model will use its own case study to show the uses and limitations of the particular approach, but where appropriate, interconnections will be made.

Respondent or classical conditioning

CASE STUDY 5.1: MRS JENNINGS AND MRS RONSON

Mrs Jennings had been diagnosed as suffering from Alzheimer's disease two years ago. The diagnosis and the forgetfulness she was experiencing caused her a great deal of anxiety. She became tearful and distraught when she lost or misplaced everyday items, or forgot the names of her grandchildren. Her next-door neighbour, Mrs Ronson, had known Mrs Jennings for over twenty years. They were close friends. Mrs Ronson visited daily and undertook many of the household and domestic tasks that Mrs Jennings found difficult. Unfortunately, Mrs Jennings began to give up trying to complete tasks that she found hard, and came to rely more and more upon Mrs Ronson. Mrs Ronson said that she felt obliged to take on more of Mrs Jennings domestic tasks because: 'It's that disease. She can no longer do anything.'

Mrs Ronson became over-stressed with the pressures of running two homes and seeing her friend of many years deteriorate in so many ways. She called the local health and social services team for people with dementia and requested help with Mrs Jennings's care.

The model and approach

Respondent or classical conditioning developed from Pavlov's famous study of dogs (Pavlov, 1927). The basic elements of the theory state that an automatic or unconditioned response may be repeated if its trigger or stimulus is paired with another event or stimulus. This 'conditioned stimulus' or trigger event may also be paired with another event to produce the original response, and so on (see Figure 5.1).

Behaviours are prompted by association with a certain event or stimulus. The same response may occur when the initial prompt is associated with a second event or stimulus. Respondent conditioning is so called because the behaviour is considered to be a response to the initial stimulus.

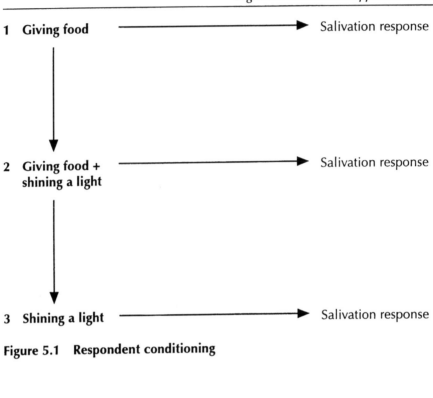

1 Giving food ———————————————► Salivation response

**2 Giving food +
    shining a light** ————————————► Salivation response

3 Shining a light ———————————► Salivation response

Figure 5.1   Respondent conditioning

Unconditioned Stimulus ——————► Unconditioned Response

Unconditioned Stimulus + ——————► Conditioned Response
Conditioned Stimulus

Conditioned Stimulus – – – – – – – – – Unconditioned Response
                                       (eventually disappears without
                                       paired Unconditioned Stimulus)

Figure 5.2   Classical extinction

If the conditioned stimulus is repeated over time without the correspond-ing appearance of the *unconditioned stimulus* or trigger, it eventually disap-pears (see Figure 5.2). Having said this, however, it must be noted that well-established phobic responses do become very resistant to change or, as it is termed in this theory, to *classical extinction*.

Respondent learning theory has been extremely helpful in explaining the development of fear reactions or phobic responses (Watson and Raynor, 1920; Sheldon, 1982, 1995; Hudson and Macdonald, 1986).

Social workers using respondent conditioning attempt to replace the fear-provoking and negative associations with more positive and pleasant ones, a process sometimes referred to as *counterconditioning*.

If, through experience, a person learns that there is no reliable connection between a stimulus event and a behaviour, this can lead to apathy and a lack of motivation. The work of Seligman (1975) on the concept of *learned helplessness* and Lefcourt (1976) and Rotter et al. (1972) is useful here. Where people are prevented from assuming control over events and their lives because they believe from experience they have no such control or influ-ence, a behavioural approach can help to re-establish some sort of order and predictability. It teaches and fosters a reassertion of control over the environment. In this sense the behavioural approach using respondent con-ditioning seeks to empower people and increase their choices in living, and is not restrictive and dogmatic in the kinds of behaviour it seeks to teach (see Case study 5.2).

CASE STUDY 5.2: MRS JENNINGS AND MRS RONSON

As well as the practical support put in, the social worker undertook a full assessment of the situation and planned with Mrs Jennings and Mrs Ronson short steps and tasks aimed at restoring some of the functioning she had lost. This gave her an increased sense of control, some measure of self-esteem and helped to lessen the fears and anxieties a little. It also gave her a sense of being in control of her life and its direction.

It had become the norm for Mrs Jennings to see her neighbour and to ask her to put on the kettle for a cup of tea. Mrs Jennings had come to rely on her neighbour for drinks in this way. They planned with the social worker to use this situation to prompt a joint effort towards making a cup of tea. Mrs Ronson, the neighbour, was extremely important here.

It was also important to provide Mrs Ronson with the capacity to con-tinue caring for Mrs Jennings. She was under increasing stress and pres-sure. This was palpable when she went to Mrs Jennings's house. She had begun to associate her shortness of breath and shaking with visiting. The social worker helped her to relax, to breathe out deeply and slowly when feeling under stress. She practised this on her own until she felt relaxed and

calm. Mrs Ronson then used this when visiting Mrs Jennings. She remarked to the social worker that she felt much better and able to cope. She no longer felt breathless and about to panic.

Activity 5.1

Read the following case vignette and suggest ways in which you might understand the situation in terms of respondent conditioning. How might you change the triggers?

Nanette moved into sheltered accommodation after being burgled by two men who also assaulted her. The experience had shaken her confidence in living alone, and her son, who had become increasingly concerned for her safety, arranged for a move to a new sheltered complex. The accommodation was supervised by an on-site warden, and Nanette received two daily checks at least. She settled in well until she noticed one day that her purse had gone missing. It was found by the warden pushed down the back of her settee. From that time on she refused to have the warden visit, and made a variety of accusations against her of stealing. The warden was aggrieved by these suggestions, and when Nanette got her up one morning at three o'clock to tell her that her mother was in her bedroom she took steps to have 'this malicious woman' removed.

Comment

At first you may think it possible to link Nanette's fear to the crime she experienced. This may well be the case, but we cannot be sure. However, it does seem that the warden had associated the accusations with malice. This was associated with Nanette's disorientation and, in fact, whatever she did it was interpreted as being intentional against the warden.

Understanding the situation in this way may not lead to a traditional behavioural intervention, but it may be especially helpful to educate the warden about dementia and about caregiving approaches. If she were to respond differently to the trigger events – the accusations, the disorientation – she may perceive Nanette in a different light.

Respondent conditioning represents one way in which we learn to behave and respond to the world around us. It is very simple, and perhaps
leaves out many of the complexities that build together to influence the
ways we respond. Other theories also have something to offer to our understanding. In the next section we shall consider operant conditioning.

Operant or instrumental conditioning

CASE STUDY 5.3: MARY AND HER SISTER
Mary lives with her sister. They are both in their eighties and have lived
together since childhood. For two years Mary has been significantly impaired in her hearing and vision. Whilst her sister describes her as being 'no
trouble most of the time', she has also discussed her concern that Mary
sometimes shouts and calls for her mother 'at all times of the day and
night'. Mary's sister says that the only thing to comfort her is either to
cuddle up on the settee together, or if it is night, for her to get into bed with
Mary.

Model and approach

Operant learning theory states that behaviours are learnt and repeated
because of the consequences immediately following their expression. The
strength, frequency and type of these consequences greatly influence any
future expression of the preceding behaviour. In respondent conditioning it
is the initial stimulus that leads to the expression of a behaviour. This is
where operant conditioning differs: it is the consequences of a behaviour
that *reinforce* it or make it more likely to recur.

Specific stimuli do not automatically elicit operant behaviour, but events
and social contexts are important as they provide cues for the kind of
behaviour that is appropriate. These cues are referred to as *antecedent stimuli*
(see Figure 5.3). Social cues can often indicate when reinforcement may be
available for the expression of a particular form of behaviour. If a practitioner can learn what signals or cues precede particular behaviours, intervention can be aimed at modifying these.

CASE STUDY 5.4: MARY AND HER SISTER
It is possible to make a beginning hypothesis in respect of Mary. The hypothesis, of course, is just that, and needs testing out. It may be that for long
periods, because she is 'no trouble', it is easy for Mary's sister to get on with
other things and possibly leave Mary out, since she can not hear the world

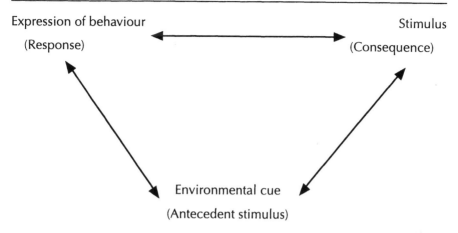

Figure 5.3   **Operant learning theory**

around her nor see what is happening. This could be an environmental cue of antecedent. At this point Mary behaves in a way that will produce desired consequences for her – she shouts and screams until physical reassurance is given. There may be other hypotheses that can be made. It is important to analyse the behaviour carefully, identifying patterns and checking out the hypotheses that have been made.

Components of operant conditioning

In order to describe operant conditioning more fully it is necessary to consider some of the various components of the theory, such as:

- types of reinforcement – what it is that maintains behaviours
- schedules of reinforcement – how these are delivered
- the controversial subject of punishment
- the shaping and moulding of behaviour
- fading.

There are a variety of types of reinforcement, or consequences which strengthen behaviours. These include:

- positive reinforcement
- negative reinforcement
- conditioned reinforcers
- generalised reinforcers
- extinction.

These are described in more detail in Box 5.1.

Box 5.1   Types of reinforcement

Positive reinforcement is something which increases the frequency and likelihood of future behaviour, and thereby strengthens it. *Negative reinforcement*, on the other hand, refers to the removal of an unpleasant stimulus or consequence when one behaves in a certain way or performs a certain action.

A *conditioned reinforcer* describes the process by which anything regularly associated with the reinforcement of behaviour eventually acquires an independent reinforcement value of its own. When the conditioned reinforcer strengthens several types of behaviour in several situations, it is known as a *generalised reinforcer*.

Extinction refers to the withholding of positive reinforcement for a behaviour which one wishes to discourage. That is, one gives no response and ignores the behaviour altogether.

Reinforcement is seldom a simple process. Human behaviour can be extremely complicated. What acts as a reinforcer for one can represent the antecedent (trigger) or the behaviour of another. The situation and its complexity can be multiplied many times within families, groups and society. The task of the social work practitioner is to break down, assess and analyse the way certain things or situations act as reinforcers, and the various functions the behaviours possess.

When designing a programme to increase or decrease behaviour, it is important to pay attention to the ways in which reinforcement is given. This is especially the case when the person at the centre of the programme has difficulties communicating their likes and dislikes and it is difficult to discern what would be a suitable reinforcer (Parker, 1995). There are a number of schedules available for use. These are shown in Box 5.2.

It is essential to make sure that the most appropriate form of reinforcement is chosen. Asking people for likes and dislikes, asking caregivers and observing people in context will provide valuable information here. It is often the case that where there is little consistency in application of a behavioural programme and the person believes there may be a chance of gaining their desired reward or reinforcement, the behaviour remains and is not easily changed. When deciding on reinforcement it is important to note that resistance to extinction remains the same for unwanted behaviours that are subject to variable-ratio schedules.

Box 5.2   Schedules of reinforcement

With *continuous reinforcement*, every occurrence of the target behaviour or that which is desired is reinforced. The aim is to establish agreed behaviours. However, behaviours reinforced in this way are easily extinguished on the withdrawal of the reinforcement. In order to maintain the behaviour, therefore, a different approach must be supplemented.

A *fixed-ratio schedule* indicates the number of responses that have to occur before reinforcement is given. An example of this would be a piecework system whereby one is paid for a certain amount of items produced, or a token economy system. Put simply, this refers to the giving of a token every time a desired behaviour is expressed. After an agreed number of these tokens have been given, the person receives the actual reward or consequence. Fixed-ratio schedules can have the effect of speeding up a response.

One of the most commonly used forms of reinforcement programme is that of *differential reinforcement*. This refers to the continuous reinforcement of one behaviour, and the *extinction* or withdrawal of positive reinforcement for another, unwanted, behaviour.

There are two main types of *intermittent schedules of reinforcement*:

1   ratio schedules – such as fixed-ratio schedules.
2   interval schedules – in which the reinforcement is given after a certain length of time has elapsed.

By far the most effective and powerful schedules of reinforcement are variable-ratio schedules. They maintain behaviours and are also very resistant to extinction. Reinforcement is given for an average but variable number of responses. The excitement derives from the unpredictability of the reinforcement.

Punishment is controversial but deserves a mention. It does not necessarily imply retribution or punitive measures as generally understood. There are two basic types of punishment:

- *Positive punishment* refers to the application of an aversive stimulus as a consequence of behaving in a certain way. The intention is to decrease the probability of the response being exhibited in the future
- *Negative punishment* refers to the withdrawal of positive reinforcement when the behaviour you wish to change is expressed.

Positive punishment, the authors believe, should not be used. Negative punishment should only be used as part of a differential programme of reinforcement. There are a number of very practical reasons for this (see Box 5.3).

Box 5.3   Factors against the use of punishment

- It leads to escape behaviour
- It may give rise to revenge and challenging behaviour
- It gives no guidance as to what is desirable behaviour, or what it is that is expected
- It acts as a general behavioural suppressant
- It has only short-term effects
- People using punishment may find it more difficult to use positive reinforcement, and punishment becomes the 'normal' response.

Some of the techniques used to 'shape' and 'chain' behaviour are similar to task-centred practice. By the selective reinforcement of certain features of behavioural performance or responses occurring at a certain level, the response can be altered gradually. The systematic and incremental shaping of behaviours by reinforcement can increase desired responses.

CASE STUDY 5.5: MRS JENNINGS AND MRS RONSON

Mrs Jennings had been experiencing difficulties in getting the sequence of dressing correct. She often put on her cardigan before her blouse and put on a pair of trousers and a dress. Mrs Ronson was upset and frustrated by this and had taken to dressing her. She did not like doing this, and Mrs Jennings also felt frustrated. A programme designed to restore self-esteem and competence at dressing was designed. This comprised a step-by-step approach to dressing, with the successful completion of each stage being rewarded. The rewards were firstly either a cup of tea or a boiled sweet. These were chosen by Mrs Jennings.

The programme designed began as follows:

Week One:

Mrs Ronson will assist with Mrs Jennings getting dressed each morning. The routine will be recorded.

Week Two:

Days one, two and three: Mrs Jennings will complete getting dressed by putting on her cardigan. When she does this, Mrs Ronson and Mrs Jennings will have a cup of tea.

Days four, five and six: Mrs Jennings will complete getting dressed by buttoning her blouse and putting on her cardigan. After this, they will have a cup of tea.

Mrs Jennings was encouraged to put on her clothes in the correct sequence, starting from the last item and taking this back to the first. In this way she achieved her goal each time and was reinforced by her success in putting on at least the final item.

In this case it was important to have the continued support and assistance of Mrs Ronson. Mrs Jennings needed encouragement and some prompting at times. The effects were wider than simply achieving a desired goal, however. Mrs Jennings felt better and was pleased that she had achieved a degree of 'independence'.

'Fading' describes the process by which control of a sequence of behaviour is gradually shifted from one set of reinforcers to another. The gradual fading of 'artificial' positive reinforcement is necessary so as not to lose the benefits by satiation, and to bring learnt, adaptive behaviour under the control of naturally occurring reinforcers. This is very important to the maintenance of adaptive behaviour.

CASE STUDY 5.6: MRS JENNINGS AND MRS RONSON

As Mrs Jennings began to regain competence in dressing, the tangible rewards she had been receiving were paired more and more with praise and encouraging comments. Although the skills she had regained needed continual reward and rehearsal, it was possible to replace the reward, to a large extent, with these more 'natural' reinforcers.

Activity 5.2

Read the following case vignette and suggest ways in which you could work positively to change the situation.

James attended a local day centre. After lunch each day he would have a short rest. Just before the afternoon's activities started, he tended to urinate in his chair. This created huge demands on staff time and took away from the activities that were planned.

Comment

First of all you would seek to assess the situation. This would involve looking in detail at the events leading up to his urinating in his chair, and comparing these with alternatives. You would also look very carefully at what happened after the event. Who did what, when and where?

You may find that there is a pattern to the behaviour. Let us imagine for a moment that he is not resting but simply quiet and bored. By urinating he manages to get considerable one-to-one attention and gains a sense of control. This may be very reinforcing and lead to the formation of a habitual response to boredom. In order to change the situation you may do two things: increase the attention he gets at certain points of the day, and ensure that any response when he urinates is matter-of-fact and does not positively reinforce. Providing stimulation and attention which is more reinforcing for him over lunchtime may decrease the behaviour.

Modelling, vicarious or imitative learning

CASE STUDY 5.7: JOYCE

Mrs Joyce Rowland was asked to stand as chairperson by a local voluntary body for people caring for those with dementia. She had been involved with the charity before her husband was diagnosed with Alzheimer's disease seven years ago. Mrs Rowland knew the workings and operations of the charity very well. She had been involved in most aspects of its organisation. However, when it came to standing for the role of chairperson she felt she did not have the skills, knowledge or intellect and declined.

Throughout her life Mrs Rowland had been content to be led by others and felt comfortable when asked to undertake a specific task, but not if asked to take responsibility. Her husband managed their affairs in a similar way to how her father had managed affairs at home with her and her mother. The fact that she had learned to handle money, insurance, bills and income tax returns gave her little belief in her ability to do things.

Model and approach

Many of our socialised behavioural tendencies are acquired by social imitation or through observation of the behaviour of others. For instance, the development of our speech patterns and the idiosyncrasies of speech in particular, such as dialect and slang, derive from our contact with and imitation of those around us. The way we use our interpersonal skills differs from culture to culture and is learnt through our observation of others around us. How to act appropriately in social situations and settings can also be explained by reference to imitative learning. This is important when considering how someone 'learns' to act in residential care, how they respond to those around them and how behaviour changes according to setting and treatment by others.

The basic components of modelling are as follows:

- *A* sees *B* performing a behaviour, and attends to *B*'s actions
- *A* forms an opinion about how this behaviour is done
- *A* notes the situation in which the behaviour was performed, and the consequences for *B*
- *A* reproduces the behaviour according to his or her perception of it (see Hudson and MacDonald, 1986).

There are a number of components necessary for modelling to be successful. It is necessary for the model to be attractive in some way to the observer, and the behaviour is more likely to be imitated if it is rewarded. Some similarity between the model and the subject is necessary, and in order to establish the behaviour within the repertoire of the subject, the opportunity to practise it and to experience positive reinforcement for doing so is needed. The success of modelling is dependent on the degree to which it creates or strengthens feelings of self-efficacy (see Box 5.4). The most powerful means of increasing this is through successful accomplishment or performance.

Box 5.4   Outcome and efficacy expectations

Bandura (1977) identifies two sets of expectations influencing what people do: *outcome expectations* and *efficacy expectations*. Outcome expectations relate to the belief that a certain behaviour will produce certain outcomes. Efficacy expectations refer to the belief that an individual has the capability to successfully produce the behaviour necessary for achieving a specified outcome.

That cognitive factors have a place in learning has long been recognised. Kelly's personal construct theory (Kelly, 1955), and the subsequent framing of social learning theory by Rotter et al. (1972), Lefcourt (1976) and Bandura (1977) provides ample evidence of this. Our cognitions, thought processes and perceptions act as mediators between environmental stimuli and consequent behaviour. People interpret the world with reference to their experiences and by watching the way other people behave. They then imitate or model a response based on these observations. Interpretations lead to expectations that certain results will result from certain courses of action in particular situations.

Sheldon (1982, 1995) outlines a number of stages involved in the modelling process. These comprise:

- identifying specific new behaviours to be learnt
- dividing the target responses into their component parts
- demonstrating competent performance
- rehearsing performance of simple sequences, shaping and correcting as required
- chaining these sequences together
- attending to matters of discrimination, when and where the behaviour is appropriate
- introducing difficulties that may be faced in real life
- supervising real-life practice and setting practical assignments.

In modelling, reinforcement can be anticipated and cognitively mediated. One can think about acting in a certain way, and about what the likely feelings would be when reinforcement occurs. Modelling is most useful in the following situations:

- where behavioural deficits are present
- in reducing interfering anxieties
- to re-establish lost behaviours.

CASE STUDY 5.8: JOYCE

Joyce Rowland felt at first that she did not have the skills and ability to fulfil the role of chair, but she was interested in doing the job. A plan of action was decided upon. She was to shadow the existing chair for six months while taking on increasing responsibility. This helped to increase her belief in her capacity to undertake the job. It also worked because of her respect for the existing chairperson and the importance of the job for her.

A modelling approach was used by the group to help her gain experience. The roles and tasks of the post were audited by Mrs Rowland and the existing chairperson, and they set these out in order of priority. She was allowed to observe the work for two meetings, and then took on limited roles and tasks to build her confidence ready for assuming the chair.

It may be argued that the uses of modelling for people with dementia are limited. The cognitive deficits and impaired capacity for learning from the example of others are restricted. However, each individual has a different capacity, and for some an image or perception of a behaviour may trigger the adoption of certain routines and behaviour in lieu of expected rewards. It is unlikely to be systematically employed in most circumstances, and its potential is therefore limited. It is seen to have effects in encouraging participation in group activities such as reminiscence groups, musical afternoons and general social events. The enjoyment of others is regarded as a powerful reinforcer, and encouraging and facilitating participation can restore or foster a tremendous feeling of self-esteem and enjoyment.

Another example of the use of modelling in social care work where dementia is an issue is found in its use with carers. Carers can receive support, help and advice from seeing the efforts and performances of other carers. Worthwhile and attractive images of caring can be adopted by carers to aid their tasks. For the social work and social care practitioner it is important to be able to determine with carers what it is they want to be able to do, and the reasons for this wish. Following this the practitioner can help break down the goal into feasible and manageable steps and encourage rehearsal. Homework and real-life practice can be set for further discussion and 'fine-tuning'.

Activity 5.3

How might you use modelling to re-establish social and interpersonal skills for a person with dementia whose confidence and opportunities for practice have diminished?

Comments

In any modelling situation it is very important to ensure that the person finds the behaviour set as a goal valuable and worthwhile. For instance, there would be little point in trying to help someone relearn using a knife and fork if throughout his or her life they had eaten using only a fork. Also, it is important that the model is respected.

It may be possible to think of situations in day and residential care in which a respected and liked member of staff can demonstrate the steps involved in holding a conversation, in laying a table, in clearing pots. In a more formal and agreed way, these can be practised and steadily built upon by the person with dementia.

It would be worthwhile spending some time in your work considering the possible opportunities for using modelling approaches, although perhaps these would be best used as part of a joint programme with the operant strategies.

Cognitive-behavioural learning

CASE STUDY 5.9: MELANIE AND HER PARENTS

Melanie Fisher had lived with her parents since returning from teacher training college thirty years ago. She cared for her mother and father as they became increasingly frail. Her mother, Mrs Fisher, was a non-insulin-dependent diabetic and had Alzheimer's disease. Mr Fisher was mentally agile but was often short of breath, very tired and unable to help with practical tasks.

Melanie had recently taken early retirement from her job in a local primary school. She felt under pressure at home, and her physical health was suffering. She thought that leaving work would make the job of caring easier.

After six months, Melanie found she could not manage. Her mother was quite a large woman and needed increased physical attention. This was difficult for Melanie, whose shoulder was weak and who felt dispirited. Social services had offered night-sitting support and a morning call to help with dressing and bathing. This relieved some of the pressure, but when she was found by the doctor in tears and shaking after straining to pick up her mother from the bathroom floor it became apparent that she could no longer continue in this way.

No further community services were found, but a residential option for both Mr and Mrs Fisher was possible, and they both wanted to try this. This was arranged. Melanie, however, felt very guilty about the move. This was exacerbated when her brother, who lived away, told her she should have looked after her parents at home.

Model and approach

Cognitive-behavioural learning theory follows on logically from modelling or imitative learning. The interpretation and evaluation of an event can be different from person to person. This in turn can lead to different emotional and behavioural responses. Where beliefs are unrealistic or particularly negative, emotional disorders can result. These beliefs are usually framed in very extreme terms and have the effect of hindering adaptive or desired goal achievement.

The cognitive-behavioural model developed to a large extent from Bandura's theory of self-efficacy (Bandura, 1977), and as a result of increasing interest in the concept of self-control (Hawton et al., 1989). This concept has three stages:

1　self-observation.
2　self-evaluation.
3　self-reinforcement.

The first wholly cognitive-behavioural approach was seen in Meichenbaum's self-instructional training (Meichenbaum, 1975). The theoretical base was simple and was clearly associated with operant thinking. Behaviour change could be facilitated by the adoption of more adaptive self-talk.

Albert Ellis, the pioneer of rational-emotive therapy, had already formulated a model for understanding the relationship between thinking and the emotions (see Box 5.5). This also added to the development of cognitive-behavioural methods.

Box 5.5   The rational-emotive model

The *A*ctivating event leads to a behavioural *C*onsequence, whilst the emotional consequences are mediated by *B*eliefs.

A belief (*B*) is:
1   an inference about the activating event (*A*);
2   an evaluation of the activating event.

A consequence (*C*) can be:
1   emotional;
2   behavioural.

The social worker's task in cognitive-behavioural work includes challenging, testing and contradicting unrealistic or negative thinking and replacing it with more adaptive cognitive inferences or evaluations.

A more sophisticated cognitive-behavioural approach has been provided by Beck (1970, 1976). This advanced and built upon the work of Ellis. Initially, the approach was applied solely to depression (Beck, 1967). The concept of depression was reframed. Negative thinking was not considered simply to be a symptom, but to be integral to the maintenance of the depression. Therefore, treatment was based upon the identification and modification of negative thoughts.

Negative thinking was construed as originating in earlier formulated assumptions which can function as motivators but also can make an individual vulnerable to certain events. A negatively perceived event can lead, in the light of the original assumption, to the production of *negative automatic thoughts*. These lower mood and increase the chances for a vicious circle of negative automatic thoughts to occur. This can maintain the depression. A set of *cognitive distortions* exert influence over general and day-to-day functioning.

The relevance of cognitive-behavioural approaches for people with dementia may be questioned. Their use is limited since the techniques rely upon the thinking capacities of those involved. However, Meichenbaum's self-talk and instructional techniques can be adapted for people in the initial stages of dementia, depending upon their personality and the degree and type of impairment suffered. Also, rational-emotive and cognitive-behavioural approaches can be used with great success with carers, relatives and people significant to the person with dementia.

CASE STUDY 5.10: MELANIE AND HER PARENTS

Melanie visited her parents two or three times each day. She hardly had time for anything else and felt increasingly pressured. Staff at the residential home suggested that she visit less. She confided in them that she felt guilty at 'being such a poor daughter' because she could not manage at home. They suggested she contact the social worker to talk through her feelings. She did so after a week.

The social worker explored her feelings of guilt and her belief that she was 'a poor daughter' and 'unfit to be their daughter'. Melanie was aware that she could not have continued caring at home because of her health and that her parents both agreed to the move. She was also conscious that her mother was well cared for and her father was enjoying the attention and concern shown by care home staff. This did not lessen her guilt or beliefs that she had failed them.

The social worker explored with her how the guilt and negative thoughts led to her continual visiting, her attempts to make amends and her self-critical comments which prevented her from doing anything she enjoyed. He encouraged Melanie to write down all the positive things she could think of about herself. She found this exercise extremely difficult and needed encouragement and some time to do it. Once completed, however, the positive statements were written on a card in short sentences. These were read out whenever Melanie felt guilty or that she was a bad daughter to her parents.

Over time these positive statements began to replace her negative perceptions and helped to reduce her guilt. In fact, she was able to set herself tasks such as joining a walking group and the local Women's Institute. This helped her to establish interests and to reduce the frequency of her visits. This was encouraged by her father, who had expressed his concern previously.

Activity 5.4

Think of situations in your work in dementia care in which debilitating thoughts and beliefs may hamper someone. When do you think that cognitive-behavioural techniques may be appropriate?

Comments

You may have thought of a range of situations concerning both people with dementia and their carers. You may have thought of staff in dementia care too.

It can be useful at times to work with people with dementia to build up self-esteem by developing positive ways to talk to oneself, positive statements to take into difficult situations. These may be as simple as 'I can do it' or 'I've managed to fill the kettle. I'm doing well.' By far the most valuable opportunities, however, are found with carers. There are opportunities for increasing skills and opportunities by positive self-talk, but also by challenging negative images and assumptions and allowing people to feel valued and valuable. This work is skilled and can take some time, but it is a valuable tool within the social worker's repertoire.

Discussion

Questions have been raised about the effectiveness and usefulness of the range of behavioural approaches for people with dementia. For instance, doubt is expressed whether a person with dementia can learn new material and new ways of acting, and also whether it is reasonable to consider attempting to change a person's behaviour by operant means if this is the case.

Jones and Miesen (1992) suggest that behavioural programmes are of little value for the person with dementia because of their decreased capacities for learning. However, an individual's reaction to and experience of dementia and capacity for new learning is varied. There is ample anecdotal evidence among practitioners to suggest this is the case. This is also borne out by clinical research into behavioural medicine with people with a range of neurological deficits. It is also important to remember that people do not act solely as individuals, but that we are all part of wider groups. We may be part of a family, group of friends, club or church member, part of a community and society. When we consider the manipulation of environmental cues and stimuli, possibilities for working with people with dementia and their carers are increased. It is also important to emphasise the effectiveness of these approaches – which has been validated in numerous empirical studies – and, in part arising from their effectiveness, their ethical basis. By discussing and noting these matters, this chapter will suggest that behavioural approaches are viable and useful for people with dementia.

When a person has lost the capacity to learn or relearn skills in the conventional sense, behavioural programmes may still be of benefit. Generally, people do not live as totally isolated individuals. There are often carers, services, relatives, friends and others who have some degree of contact with that person. By affecting the contingencies resulting from the interactions between these people and the person with dementia, changes in the behaviour can result. It is recognised that even in the latter stages of the disease, the quality of interactions and treatment can affect the person involved (Feil, 1982; 1993). It can increase their well-being (Kitwood and Bredin, 1992).

Although the fact that something works is not necessarily a justification for its use, it is an important consideration. If its effectiveness can be demonstrated, it can be monitored, evaluated and costed. It promotes accountable practice. This very fact accords with the principles of community care policy and legislation, and with professional ethical codes (see Box 5.6 and Parker, 1993).

Box 5.6   Ethics and behavioural approaches

The behavioural approach encourages self-control, as far as that is practicably possible (Hudson and Macdonald, 1986; Guydish and Kramer, 1982). Regaining lost skills may be possible in the early stages of the disease (Frogatt, 1988). Where this is not possible, learning on the part of carers and wider society may also enable a more positive and respectful approach to be taken.

Behavioural approaches encourage participation and negotiation. The participatory approach encourages motivation, and may therefore increase effectiveness. Choice is fundamental to acting with a sense of agency as a self-respecting adult. Whilst it may be necessary to employ the services of a relative, carer or advocate, dementia in itself is no reason to remove the choices available to others (Holden and Woods, 1988).

As a result of the negotiated and participatory nature, the approaches are characterised by clarity, honesty and being explicit. There is no room for covert goals, and the 'up-front' nature of the approaches makes understanding a greater possibility even when cognitive functions are impaired. They also help, again, in communicating with others involved in the care of the person with dementia.

We have already seen that the approaches are, to a large extent, effective. Being effective, they are powerful interventions, and therefore demand that the principles outlined are observed.

The approaches consider the whole situation and do not label the individual as the problem or as pathological in any way. Behavioural interventions seek to provide a means of controlling and altering the environment for the person. Where dementia is an issue, the individual person is often labelled as the problem, since it is an excess or deficit of their behaviour that is targeted for change. However, it is often the carers', relatives' or other workers' behaviours, interactions and responses that are maintaining the behavioural expression and thus become the target of intervention.

Behavioural approaches allow risk-taking and also attempt to give control to minimise risks. Risk-taking is part of life. Where possible, however, risks should be identified, made explicit and discussed openly to determine ways of reducing dangers and disruption to an individual's life (Wynne-Harley, 1991). Behavioural approaches seek to manipulate cues and consequences so as to allow a person to make informed choices wherever possible. Where this is no longer possible, the clarity and honesty of the approaches will seek to explain what consequences may result and what risks are acceptable or not.

Summary

Behavioural approaches are ethical, economical and effective. These characteristics may, in themselves, help persuade practitioners of their viability across a range of client groups, including people with dementia. However, since learning may take place at a much slower rate, the programme may be more intense and take place over a greater length of time than with some other client groups. The effectiveness of the approaches and the ethical commitment to increased control over life may suggest that not to employ behavioural approaches in situations where they may effect desired change may run counter to respect for the person. It may suggest differential treatment on the basis of age and disability. Behavioural approaches can give back an element of control. This in itself increases self-esteem and self-worth. The approaches are not only viable as a result of their effectiveness in achieving change, but in the value and worth they bestow upon people.

This chapter has provided a brief introduction to four major approaches to the way behaviours are learned and maintained. Using examples from practice situations, real life and combinations of people and events, the uses and possible applications of the theories have begun to be demonstrated. It is not suggested that any one of the four theories is more correct than another, but that each has much to offer in its explanatory and predictive power for social work practice. Where dementia is concerned, however, it must be acknowledged that those theories that rely on an approach rooted in thinking, problem-solving and cognitive ability have less to offer the person with dementia than theories relating to environmental manipulation.

6   Task-centred practice

Introduction

The task-centred approach is a logical extension of crisis intervention, although a joining of the two approaches has been challenged (Coulshed, 1991). After successfully resolving an immediate crisis, however, further beneficial changes can be achieved by working in partnership with the service user to resolve other areas of concern. Whilst partnership is stressed, task-centred practice can be used with involuntary clients and with clients whose capacity to make agreements is limited. The emphasis is upon small, achievable targets and goals, and can involve whole families or wider groups in selecting, prioritising and working towards the achievement of these. It is therefore appropriate in many circumstances for work with people with dementia, but there does need to be a clear commitment to ethical principles which protect people from the whims of others.

This chapter will review the development of task-centred practice in social work, present a basic task-centred model for social work practice, debate this within the context of Case study 6.1, and summarise the main elements of a task-centred model for people with dementia.

CASE STUDY 6.1: IRENE
Irene Maine spent a brief spell in hospital after receiving a severe electric shock from her kettle. She recovered quickly from the physical injuries she received, although she was left with a very stiff shoulder and impaired arm movement, but her confidence was considerably affected. She did not feel she could return to her house immediately because, she said, she would be afraid of making cups of tea, using any of the household implements and

generally carrying out day-to-day tasks. Two years prior to this accident she had suffered a stroke which had left her speech and memory damaged.

For a short while her son took her into his home and family. This did not work well, and he called social services for help in finding his mother somewhere more suitable to stay. Irene was adamant that she would not enter residential care, but felt uncomfortable at the prospect of returning home. The social worker undertook an assessment of her needs and those of her family. Together with the family, the social worker planned a range of options they could pursue to allow her the freedom and security she wanted and to ensure that any risks were minimised.

The model and approach

Task-centred work is associated with problem-solving, behavioural social work and crisis intervention (Howe, 1987). In the most simply stated terms, task-centred practice refers to the chaining of a series of incremental steps designed to achieve goals which have been agreed between the service user and practitioner (Doel and Marsh, 1992). Task-centred practice is about purposeful actions. Social work practitioners will have heard the term frequently and may have their own ideas about what constitutes task-centred work. The work is time-limited, structured and problem-focused. It is an active collaboration between practitioner and service user.

The development of task-centred practice

Alongside growing dissatisfaction with open-ended psychodynamic approaches to social work in the 1960s, an increasing emphasis was placed upon the participation of the client. Client self-determination and a concern to increase client motivation in the intervention process began to exert an influence on practice. In this context Perlman (1957, 1986) emphasised the problem-solving approach to social work. This was heavily influenced by ego psychology, but was distinguished from traditional casework approaches because it dealt with the client's presenting problems. Perlman's work constituted an influential forerunner of problem analysis within task-centred work.

In 1969, Reid and Shyne examined the relative merits of brief and long-term social work. This was a novel approach, and a particular treatment strategy was developed which emphasised:

- focusing on the key aspect of the problem
- collaborating with the client and developing open, honest, and explicit objectives

- reviewing goals and objectives to check achievements
- paying attention to the way families can generalise their learning for future use.

The principal findings of this research indicated that brief, active treatment led to more progress during contact, and that benefits were just as durable six months after the work had ended.

It was thought that brief intervention affected the workers in the level and timing of their activity, in the feasibility of goals and in planning, motivation and performance.

The nature and level of worker activity required greater specification and clarity. Also, the timing of the activity occurred much earlier on in the work, when – as noted for crisis intervention – possibilities for change may be greater. Whilst the action focus and specification by worker may have conveyed a positive message to clients, the planned ending was thought to have raised the motivation to work and provided a sense of accomplishment where successful small-task accomplishment had been achieved.

The task-centred practice model developed from this initial research (Reid and Epstein, 1972). At first a seven-point typology of problems was presented for which task-centred work may be effective:

1   interpersonal conflict.
2   dissatisfaction in social relations.
3   relations with formal organisations.
4   role performance.
5   social transition.
6   reactive emotional distress.
7   inadequate resources.

This was quickly extended to include any other psychological or behavioural problem not specified in the original list (Reid, 1978). Doel and Marsh (1992) simplify this list by suggesting that task-centred work deals with 'social difficulties' agreed by service user and practitioner or recognised by others such as the courts. This provides a useful understanding which is easily transferable to all settings in which social workers are involved.

Initially, task-centred work developed in the USA, but there were growing concerns for an ethical, efficient and effective intervention in British social work (Goldberg and Connelly, 1981; Sheldon, 1986; Macdonald and Sheldon, 1992). The client perspective, as reported by Mayer and Timms (1970), demonstrated a need to develop interventions that were perceived as effective by those using social work services. Emphasis on user perspectives has grown and developed in importance (Cheetham et al., 1992).

The development of task-centred social work practice owes a great deal to the positive features associated with it, which comprise:

- the specificity and clarity of its aims and purpose
- the contractual agreement between worker and client
- the concentration upon achievable goals
- its time-limited nature
- the task-oriented focus and structured sequential approach
- its reported effectiveness and measurability.

Some social workers, however, have been too ambitious in setting goals and objectives. This has been the case for people with dementia and may have led to practitioners abandoning a potentially useful interventive strategy. In practice, it is essential to work towards small, incremental but achievable goals if the work is to be successful. Doel (1994) has emphasised the core values of partnership and empowerment underpinning task-centred approaches. Clients are seen as those who know best about the situations they face:

The success of the task-centred approach is based on the simple idea that small successes build confidence and self-esteem, and that people are more likely to

---

Activity 6.1

What benefits and limitations does the task-centred model have for people with dementia and their carers?

Comments

You may have suggested that the clarity, specificity and practical nature of the model can offer benefits to people dealing with losses of skills and taking on new roles in caregiving. Its structure and goal-oriented purpose is clear, and this may provide additional benefits in keeping on track and setting simple task sequences for people with memory problems.

You may, however, have suggested that the learning difficulties associated with dementia prevent its use because once one task is completed the person with dementia cannot make the link to the next stage. In fact, all people with dementia are different and have different capacities for new learning. Also, there is an emphasis in task-centred work on small and feasible goals. This is often forgotten by social workers.

achieve these successes if they are working towards something they have chosen to do. The task-centred worker helps people to make choices about what they want to do. Central to this idea is the belief that, by and large, people are capable of reasoning and that they are the best people to make these choices. (Doel, 1994, p. 22)

It is therefore important to work with a clear, planned and structured model which is grounded in the values of respect for people and their choices. It is to such a model for practice that we will now turn.

A model for practice

Doel (1994) states that the task-centred approach is unusual in its emphasis on the practical, but believes it has clear links with learning theories. The achievement of tasks and goals can be very strongly reinforcing – in fact, it is this that increases client motivation. Gambrill (1994) argues that the task-centred model draws heavily upon behavioural methods, but then rejects the theoretical and conceptual underpinnings associated with it.

The following model will compare the original approach with two others developed for social work in the UK (see Box 6.1). The models are comparable in general terms, and simply emphasise different aspects of the process. For instance, Doel (1992, 1994) makes the important point that the social worker must carefully consider the mandate for work to be done so as to ensure that authority is employed correctly and appropriately prior to intervention. This process assists in establishing clarity. Legal obligations are made explicit, as are the purposes of the service user and practitioner in using the method.

There is a general agreement on the stages and processes involved in task-centred work (see Box 6.2).

Task-centred practice is, as we have mentioned earlier, a problem-solving approach to social work. As a result, the exploration, identification, specification and prioritisation of a problem to work upon is fundamental to the model. All models debate at some point the formulation of an agreement between service users and practitioners, but there is considerable debate whether this agreement should be written or remain verbal. The action focus is central to the model and process. This includes planning and agreeing tasks, specifying roles and responsibilities, completing agreed tasks, reviewing achievements and modifying planning. Although an element of review is included at each stage, the final session is devoted to an overall review of the accomplishments of the service user. We shall now explore this model in greater detail.

Box 6.1 Models of task-centred social work practice

	Reid and Epstein (1972)	Payne (1991)	Doel and Marsh (1992)
			Mandate for the work
	Identification of the target problem	Problem specification	Exploring problems
Stage/ Process		Contract negotiation	Written agreement
	Task formulation	Planning of tasks	Tasks – planning and implementation
	Task implementation	Task implementation	
	Continual assessment		
	Ending	Ending	Ending

Box 6.2 The main features of task-centred models

Stage	Process
Problem stage	Exploration and assessment process
Agreement stage	Negotiation and specification of the purpose of the work
Task stage	Planning and implementation
Ending stage	Review of work done, change achieved, processes involved

Problem stage

The initial assessment focuses on the reasons for the practitioner's involvement, the wants and wishes of the service users, and begins to create a sharper focus to the work. Doel and Marsh (1992) use the metaphor of a newspaper to describe the process. First of all a broad-sweep approach is taken to problem identification – this is somewhat akin to glancing at the front page of the newspaper to gain a broad understanding of what is happening. To gain greater detail and clarity, one might search the headlines, identify lead stories and then turn to the inside story that sparks most interest.

The identification of problems is a joint venture in which service users are encouraged to describe problems as they see them. These are then placed in some kind of order, practitioners check their understanding, and construct an initial problem profile with service users and others to gain corroborative information. At this stage a rank order can be drawn up and agreement reached on the priority problem to be worked upon.

Once the profile of problems has been prioritised, the target problem can be described in precise detail. The process is the same in terms of negotiating, checking understanding, reaching agreement and specifying as exactly as possible what the problem is (see Box 6.3).

Box 6.3   The problem exploration process

- Identify the broad range of potential problems
- Reach tentative agreement and develop a problem list
- Challenge problems which cannot be changed or resolved
- Seek the views of others in the construction of a more detailed problem profile
- Seek precise details of the problem – when, where, what, how, frequency?
- Specify the problem in clear and explicit behavioural terms.

This stage demands clear listening and interview skills on the part of the practitioner. Gaining, categorising and checking information is not easy, especially if the service user finds it difficult to communicate, internalise new information or concentrate. However, it is useful to 'widen the net' at this stage and to include family members, other carers and advocates. This can help elicit useful information and to identify problems which are meaningful to the family or environment in which the person with dementia lives, but there are dangers in relying on the views of others. Having access to articulate carers and relatives is no substitute for consulting the person with dementia as fully as possible. The exploration process can be seen as a funnel (see Figure 6.1).

Activity 6.2

Read the following case vignette and suggest ways in which the problem exploration process may take place.

James and Edna Gardener lived on a small council estate near their daughter and her family. James had a stroke which had left him weak and unable to walk long distances. His speech was also a little slurred at times. Edna had Alzheimer's disease. She found it very difficult and very frustrating to concentrate on conversations and daily tasks. James was increasingly worried about paying the bills, especially after receiving a final demand from the gas board.

Comments

It would be easy to concentrate on James in an interview and look at his concerns about paying the bills and the final demand they had received. This would fail to take into account Edna's concerns and frustrations, and might end up increasing or exacerbating them. It may be that exploring issues together with them would highlight other concerns as the priority. For instance, it may be that the reason for not paying the bills is because of James' decreased mobility. If Edna was assisted to follow (and perhaps relearn) her way to the gas board, matters could be sorted out. This happened in a case known to one of the authors, in which the husband, a man with Alzheimer's disease, relearned the way into town following a well-known routine from earlier in his life. Through a process of working out small steps and tasks he was able to pay any bills when his wife, a woman with severe arthritis, was unable to go with him.

Using the problem-exploration questions suggested above with people with dementia and their carers will give you a view from many angles and help you to reach an agreement acceptable to all involved.

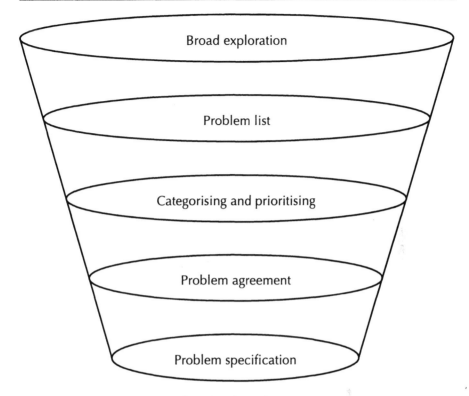

Figure 6.1 The problem exploration funnel

The agreement stage

The second stage is that of reaching an agreement. There is debate as to whether the agreement between service users and practitioners should be written or should remain oral. Whilst oral agreements can be less frightening and imposing (and are necessary where a person cannot read), a written contract or agreement adds to specificity, and can be referred to at a later date if a dispute over tasks or responsibilities arises. A written agreement can be extremely useful in establishing clear parameters for work where remembering is difficult or where there are many people involved. The process of making an agreement is shown in Box 6.4.

Reid and Epstein (1972, 1977) include priority ranking of problems, tentative identification of the target problem and greater specification in their first stage, and recommend that an explicit agreement should be made about these matters with the client.

Doel (1994) identifies three important factors to be borne in mind while attempting to delineate and agree upon goals:

Box 6.4   The agreement process

1 Select a target problem or set of problems on which to work – remember, the client defines the problem. (If choosing more than one problem, these should be set out in rank order.)
2 Decide on the desired outcome or goal of the intervention.
3 Specify the first set of tasks to meet goals.
4 Agree upon the amount of contact and duration of involvement with the practitioner.

---

1 ensuring that the goal is really what the person wants to achieve, so as to increase or maximise motivation.
2 ensuring they are feasible and achievable.
3 determining whether the goal is desirable or runs counter to agency policy or values.

Task stage

It is essential that planned tasks are explicit, are practicable for the client to undertake outside sessions, and are mutually agreed. There are two basic types of task:

- general tasks which set out the treatment policy
- operational tasks which define exactly what the client will do.

They may involve a single action or a set of actions. Tasks may be set for the client to do alone, or the client may do one task while the worker or relative does something else. They may also be shared. At this point a more specific and task-focused agreement can be negotiated (see Box 6.5).

Box 6.5   The process of making a task-focused agreement

1 Select and agree upon a target problem.
2 Decide upon the desired outcome or goal of the intervention.
3 Design a set of tasks to meet the target.
4 Agree upon the amount of contact and duration of involvement.

All work in sessions from now onwards is directed towards facilitating task achievement by the client. As the interventive process proceeds, the tasks may be revised towards greater specificity. This allows progress to be measured and the intervention to be altered to achieve the maximum gain. The social work role and the intensity of involvement depends upon the agreement, the capacity of the service user and the involvement of others who may help with the programme. This flexibility allows the model to be used with a wide range of people. The process for this stage is shown in Box 6.6.

Box 6.6   The task implementation process

- Set up a system of recording, especially when sequences or repetitions of actions are required
- Identify what needs to be done to achieve agreed tasks, how, and by whom
- Agree incentives or rewards for successful task completion
- Ensure and check out that the client understands the value of the tasks and how completing them helps to meet their agreed goals or aims
- Practice, by modelling and guided practice if necessary, the relevant skills to be learnt
- Identify any obstacles to task achievement
- Plan the worker's tasks that will contribute to the successful completion of the intervention. This may include working with other people and agencies, arranging for rewards and incentives, or sharing tasks with clients when they lack resources/ skills to do them alone.

Source: Payne (1991).

During each session, both the worker and client should review achievements jointly. Some difficulties may arise at this stage. Doel (1994) points out that the client's motivation may wane, and as a result tasks may remain unaccomplished. If practitioners identify this, they may be able to renegotiate with the client and, if necessary, modify goals. However, progress may be diverted off course by a range of other factors affecting the client, and care needs to be taken to allow a degree of flexibility in the process (Coulshed, 1991). At this stage it is useful to involve carers and relatives. This may encourage perseverance and, if the contract is written, can help to keep a focus on the agreed tasks and the goals sought.

Ending stage

It is important that the time-limited nature of the intervention is mentioned at the outset, and that the end is always in sight. This provides a focus and, hopefully, encourages the client's motivation and that of other significant people involved. The ending phase is undertaken jointly between client and worker, and includes the features set out in Box 6.7.

Box 6.7   The ending stage

- Describe the problem as it was at the outset and as it is now
- Significant participants should assess any changes made
- Plan for the future – how they will use new skills and strategies for coping
- Negotiate new contracts to carry on with any unfinished work on the initial problem or to establish a new target problem and new task definition
- Make explicit the end to a piece of work when involvement continues because of statutory obligations, residential care, etc.
- Consider a move to longer-term intervention, or referral to another agency for additional or alternative help.

Source: Payne (1991).

However carefully planned the intervention has been, the client may not wish to end contact. This may highlight a different need, and that work is needed in areas of self-confidence and efficacy, or it may indicate a need for social activities and stimulation. When the agreed goal is not achieved at the end of the planned sessions, more time may be negotiated if it is felt this will facilitate goal achievement (Doel, 1994).

Throughout the four key stages involved in task-centred practice, it is important to be both systematic and responsive (Coulshed, 1991). It is essential to be systematic so as to keep the client's focus on the task in hand, but it is also necessary to be responsive to other important factors in the life of the client. The main point is to be flexible enough to keep the client focused and to acknowledge other concerns. This is especially important in work with people with dementia, since structure can provide a sense of continuity and comfort, yet a degree of flexibility is important to deal with new situations as they arise.

The contractual basis of the work has been highlighted by some as making explicit the terms of the relationship: the unequal power relationship between practitioner and service user. It may be argued that the power imbalance that remains because of the authority vested in social workers prevents mutual co-operation (Rojek and Collins, 1987). However, the empirical base of the intervention and its proven effectiveness in meeting specific modest goals will ensure that its popularity and use continues. The strong demand for accountability, financial efficiency and effectiveness in the interventions that social workers employ makes it popular. In order to ensure that social work practitioners develop a research focus to ensure that services given to clients meet these needs, such strategies that are open to measurement are necessary.

Activity 6.3

What are the main stages involved in the task-centred way of working?

Comments

The four main stages involved are:

1 problem exploration.
2 agreement on target and setting of goals.
3 designing tasks and implementing a plan.
4 ending the work.

Task-centred work is systematic and time-limited. It is a practical way of working.

The emphasis in ending is important. This is designed to focus the mind and increase motivation. Of course, for people with dementia it may be that targets, goals and endings are forgotten. Whilst this is often used as a criticism of task-centred work for people with dementia, it can also be one of its strengths. Continual review, rehearsal and reminders of the time-limited nature help to ensure that work is completed and that dependency is avoided.

Studies concerning the use of task-centred practice

Task-centred practice is noted for its effectiveness in a wide variety of areas in social work. Positive benefits have been reported in terms of increased respect and a demystification of the social work role for clients in the study of a generic social work team by Goldberg et al. (1977). Task-centred practice has been used in social work in the treatment of child abuse (Nicol et al., 1988; Barth, 1989), with families as a whole (Reid and Helmer, 1985; Reid, 1987; Benbenishty and Ben-Zaken, 1988), with marital problems and relationships (Butler et al., 1978; Reid and Strother, 1988), in psychiatric settings (Gray, 1987; Garvin, 1992; Rabinowitz and Lukoff, 1995), in employee assistance programmes (Ramkrishnan and Balgopal, 1992), and self-harm (Butler et al., 1978; Gibbons et al., 1979).

CASE STUDY 6.2: IRENE
Whilst there was a clear legislative and agency mandate for the work with Irene following the assessment under the National Health Service and Community Care Act 1990, there was also a mandate from the wide number of significant people involved. Most notably these included her son and family and herself.

A broad problem exploration identified a need to live as independently as possible whilst being able to manage daily living tasks. Further discussion and observation including Irene and her family identified the tasks of compiling shopping lists, going to the shops and cooking as her priorities.

It was possible to identify two general goals in the subsequent agreement for work. These comprised securing alternative and suitable accommodation, and being able to budget, shop and cook for herself. The first goal lent itself to separation into targets concerning lodging an application and securing a meeting with housing representatives leading to the achievement of the final goal. The second goal of gaining independent living skills was broken down into smaller targets and tasks.

The agreement negotiated stated clearly her overall goal to achieve as great a degree of independence as possible. This resulted in agreement on the first target – gaining an independent flat in a sheltered housing scheme. The worker, Irene's son and Irene herself all had tasks to complete to achieve this target. These were written down according to responsibility, sub-tasks, dates for completion and review, the number of sessions to be held and dates for a final review of the work. The initial agreement looked as follows:

Agreement between Irene Maine, Bill and Jenny Maine, and Newtown Social Services Department

This agreement sets out the goals identified by Irene and the necessary tasks and responsibilities of each party in achieving them.

Goal:
Irene wishes to live as independently as possible. This means she needs to secure alternative accommodation and to be able to plan, shop and cook for herself.

Targets:
1 To gain independent accommodation.
2 To gain independent living skills.

Independent accommodation
The social worker will bring information concerning a range of properties available in the area. These will be discussed with Irene.

Following agreement on the type of property and area desired, the social worker will assist Irene in approaching the housing officer in order to make an application.

The social worker will seek and provide contact numbers in the housing office for Irene and the family. They will check progress weekly.

Irene's family will take her to view any property offered.

Irene and her family, with support from the social worker, will complete any necessary agreements for the housing licence once a property has been accepted.

Bob and Jenny Maine will help to move and settle Irene into the property.

Independent living skills
Jenny will assist Irene with planning a shopping list for the weekly shop.

Irene will accompany Jenny and Bob to the supermarket for the weekly shop.

Jenny will encourage Irene to make the evening meal once each week.

Signed ....

Signed ....

Signed ....

The agreement was successful, and Irene moved into a sheltered housing flat within four weeks. At this point further targets were negotiated which involved coping in this new situation. Irene had developed a fear of using the kettle and cooker after her accident. While she had lived with her son she had avoided using them and left this to her daughter-in-law, son and grandchildren. The practice undertaken in designing shopping lists, shopping and making drinks and preparing food highlighted a number of concerns. Having secured her desired level of independence, she needed to develop her skills to function at an appropriate level. How this might be achieved was discussed and agreed. This led to the introduction of a home care assistant who would break down and chain together the tasks associated with these actions in conjunction with Irene. They would then work, by modelling and encouragement, to achieve a greater degree of accomplishment and task achievement each day. The skills would be rehearsed at each session, with sessions becoming less frequent on a planned basis. The programme ran as follows:

Agreement on independent living skills

The social services department will provide a home care assistant for four weeks initially to encourage Irene to plan her meals and write a shopping list.

In the first week after moving, the home care assistant will take Irene for a walk in the area to get used to the shops and amenities.

For the first four weeks the home care assistant will accompany Irene to the shops twice each week.

The tasks involved in making a cup of tea will be practised in the first week. In the second week, making snacks and light meals will be practised. Following this, in the third and fourth weeks Irene will complete the tasks to make a full meal under the supervision of the home care assistant. (These plans are the subject of the care plan.)

After four weeks the programme will be reviewed. However, if at any time there are worries and concerns, any party to the agreement can call a meeting to discuss matters.

The review of these tasks – monitored by the home care assistant, the warden of the sheltered scheme, the family, Irene herself and the social worker – provided a clear picture of accomplishment and continuing need. With encouragement, Irene regained her confidence in completing the tasks, although it became evident that her short-term memory problems affected completion at times. This was discussed at the review, and having worked in this task-centred way throughout, the family agreed – with Irene's consent – to break down daily living tasks with her and encourage completion. Social services maintained a home care assistant to assist with shopping on a once-weekly basis.

The immediate benefit of a task-centred approach was its clarity. Although Mrs Maine herself suffered from short-term memory loss and disorientation to time and place, the explicit nature of the work allowed her to continually remind herself of its purpose, and also, importantly, to ensure that agreed and negotiated matters took precedence over issues of concern to other people involved. This helped to protect her rights.

At one point the social worker was asked by her son if greater care, and possibly residential care, could be arranged. His reasons for this were well intentioned as he wanted the best, as he saw it, for his mother. He believed that she would soon forget that she did not wish to be there and would settle in. The explicit nature of the agreement helped to remind participants of the purpose of the work and to maintain a focus.

Also, the work was empowering in that it capitalised on the strengths of the person involved, was clear and explicit and could be learned by those involved to help secure other benefits in the future without reliance on professionals.

Activity 6.4

List some of the values underpinning the task-centred approach. How do these relate to dementia care?

Comments

The emphasis on partnership, mutual agreement and action towards achieving tasks and goals demonstrates a clear concern for self-determination, self-efficacy and respect for persons. It may be argued that in dementia care the person is less able to form agreements, to work towards goals and stay on task, and is unlikely to learn from or join in the process. In practice, the person's involvement and capacity varies from individual to individual. This is also the case for people who do not have dementia.

It is important to remember that cognitive deficits and an impaired capacity for learning does not diminish the need for active involvement. In fact, the process of action towards goals may be motivating and encouraging, and may produce benefits for the person with dementia as much as the achievement of those goals.

Summary

Where short-term goals are clearly specified, achievement can be promoted and encouraged by concentration on the agreed tasks. This is particularly appropriate for people with dementia because it is simple and clear and demands a partnership which encourages attention to the task. There are, of course, difficulties in working in a task-focused way with people who find it difficult to concentrate and to relearn lost skills. Often the opportunities to do so have been denied or are simply no longer there. However, it is possible to work with larger groups of people, including family and carers, to encourage the achievement of specified tasks. Where this is possible, it can motivate others around the person with dementia, and can foster an attitude which sees the person and their dignity before the dementia.

Task-centred work is potentially a very powerful and empowering approach to social work. It does, however, have its dangers. Where the person is no longer able to make decisions and agreements or to voice wants and wishes, or is denied the opportunity, carers and relatives may, often unwittingly, voice their own needs. There is therefore a clear reason to maintain a social work involvement initially, at least, to ensure that the rights of the individual are specified and promoted.

A final benefit of this type of approach to social work with people with dementia is that it is open to scrutiny. Family, carers, the individual can all see what has been achieved and what has been agreed. This also lends itself, to agency evaluation procedures in these days of increased accountability, and to practitioner research into good practice.

7 Working with challenging behaviours

Introduction

Dealing with behaviours described as 'challenging' can be anxiety-provoking, challenging in itself, and can leave a void in one's sense of control. It raises concerns for personal safety and the safety of others because challenging behaviour is often associated with potential and actual violence, although in fact it is much more than this.

We will present here a brief description of challenging behaviour and outline three approaches that are important to effective management, personal safety and the care and quality of life of the person presenting the behaviours labelled 'challenging':

- the use of interpersonal skills
- the sensitive planning of routines, and physical environment
- positive reinforcement and behavioural approaches.

These approaches often use techniques and models already mentioned in earlier chapters. Challenging behaviour is dealt with in a separate chapter because of its importance to contemporary practice in the community, day care and residential care.

It is recognised that emergencies do occur, and situations may well develop that present an immediate physical threat to a person's safety or that of other people. This is not the focus of this chapter. These situations demand an adequate staff policy that delineates exactly what can and cannot be done in terms of restraint and protection (Seaton, 1994).

CASE STUDY 7.1: BILL AND VIOLET

Bill Sanderson lived with his second wife, Violet. They married over forty years ago after his first wife left and divorced him. They both felt punished and ostracised by relatives and friends because of the divorce. Bill was alleged to have been violent to his first wife on a regular basis, and this coloured people's response to them. As a result they kept themselves to themselves and had few friends in the area.

Bill suffered from a stroke, after which his moods began to swing from placid to upset and emotional or threatening. The doctor said this was only to be expected and she would have to get used to it. Violet was told that Bill would be likely to be upset because of the slight loss of speech and weakness in his left arm.

Prior to the stroke, Bill had begun to talk more about his first wife and how he missed her. He remembered his days in the army and his experiences at Dunkirk. He also began to look through his scrapbooks kept from the days he toured as an amateur boxer before the war. Violet was upset when he mentioned his first wife and thought he was deliberately goading her. Whenever she mentioned anything, he would snap at her and tell her not to be silly. Finally, she tried to ignore his comments, and when he began speaking about his first wife she would sit in the kitchen and listen to the radio. After the stroke, Bill seemed to retreat more into his rememberings and to be increasingly annoyed at what he saw as Violet's attempts to undermine him.

Bill was a big man, and the stroke had weakened him. Violet had to help him get up in the morning, get into bed and had to help with bathing. Bill did not like this. It frustrated him, and he shouted and swore at her. Violet also found it difficult. She was quite frail, and herself suffered from high blood pressure. Matters reached a critical point when Bill seemed to think he was back in the boxing ring and hit Violet.

She called social services for help in looking after him. Violet thought that if she could have support with getting him up, bathing and physical care, this would take the pressure off her and him, and that he would calm down. She also wanted some help in dealing with his insults and what she perceived to be his deliberate attempts to pick on her.

Models and approaches

What is challenging behaviour?

The term 'challenging behaviour' encompasses much more than physical aggression and violence, although it is these that cause most anxiety and consequently receive most attention.

'Challenging behaviour' refers to actions observable by their commission or omission, and their resulting consequences. These actions are expressed by people in a social or interactive context that they consider to present something difficult or demanding, but the 'challenge' is experienced by others, rather than the person exhibiting the behaviour. In this sense, the term 'challenging behaviour' has great value and meaning. Individuals are not labelled as problems themselves, nor are the behaviours viewed solely as problems. The challenging behaviour presents a demanding task to others involved with the person expressing the behaviour. The challenge for social work practitioners is to analyse and understand the meaning of and intention underlying the behaviour, which can lead to the design of effective interventions. The behaviours exhibited may be the only way a person has of communicating or being heard, and whilst it may not be the most desired way of communicating, it no doubt results in being heard and/or responded to.

Assessment

Any competent and effective intervention relies on a comprehensive assessment of all relevant areas of a person's life. When making an assessment of a person who is found to be challenging, the assessment is especially important since it may help to explain how that behaviour arose. This is even more the case with a person with dementia because of the cognitive impairment which may hamper that person from communicating in any other way. Each assessment should take into account:

- social and family history
- medical history
- psychiatric history
- any present medical or psychiatric conditions
- sensory impairment.

A full personal and medical history is important in the management and treatment of repeated behaviours found challenging by staff – for example, are they perhaps the result of a long-standing psychiatric disorder, a medical condition and/or pain that can not be expressed in any other way, or does the person suffer from any form of sensory impairment? However, having screened for these, strategies for the ethical and effective management of challenging behaviours are necessary. Two reasons in particular stand out: the protection and safety of staff; increasing opportunities and the social/interactive repertoire of the person exhibiting the behaviour. We now turn to strategies and management.

Activity 7.1

Can you describe what the concept of challenging behaviour means and how this relates to people with dementia?

Comments

It is useful to remember that the behaviour is challenging to those observing it, and it may serve another function for the person with dementia. It may be the only effective way he or she now has to communicate, so the task of the social worker is to work with the person to unravel the communication within the behaviour and to seek alternatives that are less challenging.

It is also important to remember that the behaviour may be a reaction to care practices that are less than helpful in promoting personhood and self-worth. We need to be able to change and alter our approaches when necessary.

Dealing with challenging behaviour

Two matters resulting from the previous discussion need to be highlighted:

- Behaviour is often a means of communication, and the individual's needs and what they are trying to communicate must be central in the minds of caring professionals
- The behaviour is a function of its environment, and individuals are not to be seen as the problem.

Box 7.1   Approaches to challenging behaviours

- the use of interpersonal skills
- an environmental approach
- positive reinforcement and behavioural approaches.

There are three main ways in which challenging behaviour can be managed (see Box 7.1), and an integration of all three may be necessary to fully and effectively deal with the individual's needs identified by the behaviour.

The use of interpersonal skills

Most violent incidents have fairly predictable antecedents, and are often preceded by verbal confrontation and high levels of arousal (McDonnell et al., 1994). Although no single particular approach has been demonstrated as entirely successful in the reduction of violent incidents, predicting the

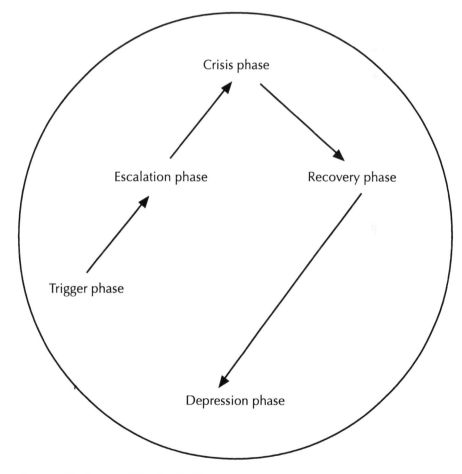

Source: Kaplan and Wheeler (1983).

Figure 7.1   The cycle of violence

incident is clearly important. Many different approaches can be used after predicting the potential situation. Kaplan and Wheeler (1983) offer a five-stage cycle to help examine potentially violent situations (see Figure 7.1). This model helps to identify trigger events and to isolate patterns which may help in designing effective ways of managing the behaviour and dealing with the underlying concerns.

McDonnell et al. (1994) describe a number of defusion strategies that rely on the use of interpersonal skills. These are illustrated in Box 7.2.

Box 7.2   Defusion strategies

- **Mood-matching** – This implies that one should match the other person's arousal level, but not his or her emotion. This is very difficult to do and may be potentially hazardous. Whilst raising one's voice may help de-escalate a potentially violent situation, it may act as a cognitive trigger to someone else
- **Surprise/shock methods** – These rely on non-physical surprises such as bellowing or making a sudden loud noise to ward off a potential attack or the use of alarms. Again, these may be perceived as a threat and need to be employed cautiously, attempting not to trigger off further potential for violence by increasing alarm and threat
- **Assertiveness training** – Whilst popular and very useful in some settings, this relies upon the notion that a person finds themselves in a potentially violent situation partly because they are ineffective in expressing their wishes. There may also be a problem distinguishing between aggression and assertion in some cases
- **Other strategies** that have been employed include physical restraint, seclusion, and self-defence training. Research evidence is ambivalent about their effectiveness, and with the first two, questions of ethics and acceptability are raised alongside the very real danger of increasing retaliatory situations
- **Interpersonal and listening skills** – Stokes (1987a, 1987b, 1987c, 1987d) provides a wealth of useful information in his four books concerning common problems in dementia. He offers a number of 'dos and don'ts' that may help in offsetting potentially violent and conflictual situations.

A fuller examination of the interpersonal skills used in social care work is important, so it may be useful to remind ourselves of the basic interpersonal skills. Attention to voice and speech is essential in ensuring you demonstrate calm and that you are no threat to the person involved, who may find the world a confusing and frightening place. Key points to remember include avoiding making judgements or using terms that might imply evaluation; using an even tone; speaking fairly slowly and clearly in a manner that demonstrates interest and concern, and being prepared to listen to justifiable complaints.

Remember also that your body language needs to be congruent with your verbal speech, since people notice discrepancies. It is important to convey a non-threatening and open stance. The frequency and intensity of your eye contact needs attention. Using eye contact can be positive, but if maintained over time it can be threatening and imply aggression, which may make the situation worse. Associated with this is the space you maintain between youself and the other person. Leave enough to ensure the person feels he/she has a route of escape and is not trapped. Doing this also helps to ensure your own safety.

Although guidelines concerning the use of interpersonal skills can be provided, they must remain only guidelines, and it needs to be remembered that there are cultural and individual differences in the use and interpretation of the way we interact.

It is important to consider how we listen to other people, especially when there is the possibility of aggression and violence. Cournoyer (1991) notes four main components of listening:

- *hearing* another's words and speech
- *observing* non-verbal gestures and positions
- *encouraging* full expression
- *remembering* what is said or communicated.

If we listen to another using these components, then we convey respect and genuine interest. This can allow a person to discuss their concerns and complaints freely, it can help elicit points and issues that raise tension and potential conflict, and can help the practitioner to calm the situation whilst dealing with whatever message is conveyed by the other person.

In order to ensure you understand what is being said, it is useful to paraphrase and reflect or mirror the communications of the other person. There are three important steps to active listening:

1 *inviting* the person to speak, or communicating interest and acceptance by your body language, speech and expression.

2 *listening* – hearing, observing, encouraging and remembering what is being communicated.

3 *reflecting* – paraphrasing what is conveyed to you.

As with all interpersonal approaches, there are some dangers. One must seek to avoid reflecting back the same words (see Nelson-Jones, 1983), reflecting too often, and interrupting frequently. These may, of course, incense the person you are listening to and lead to the expression of the very behaviour you are seeking to avoid.

An environmental approach

There needs to be a sensitive overhaul of all procedures and policies concerned with the introduction, continuation and management of personal service provision, especially when providing intimate care and intensive care in the person's home, when introducing new staff, and when facilitating a move into day care or residential care (see Stokes, 1987a, 1987b, 1987c, 1987d; Seaton, 1994; and Netton, 1993).

Routines need to be established that reflect the needs of individuals whilst providing an overall level of security and continuity. These need to be sensitively rehearsed with people, and positive encouragement needs to be given to aid learning. The vignette in Case study 7.2 illustrates this.

CASE STUDY 7.2: ARTHUR

Arthur, a placid and calm man of 86, was introduced to permanent residential care in a different home after a short period in respite care. The residential home telephoned his family and social services asking for him to be removed after four days because he was urinating in the sink, behind radiators and in the corridor. It transpired that he had not been shown where the toilet was, nor had the routine of the home been explained to him. He had changed from being mild-mannered and placid to being a distraught and aggressive man in a matter of days. With sensitive, adequate and continued explanations and reinforcement for appropriate urinating, however, he settled into the home without further incident. In the future, the home paid greater attention to introductory material and a settling-in period to help orientate new residents.

Orientating features need to be introduced into the environment (Marshall, 1997). Continuity and familiarity are important, and an environment that is not uniform and confusing is not a luxury but essential to maintaining and helping establish a sensitive, individually needs-led approach to the provision of services (Cohen and Weisman, 1991).

Reality orientation – an approach derived from behavioural models – can provide positive benefits, especially if it is undertaken on a continual basis, although being presented with a hurtful and confusing present can sometimes be very distressing, and reality orientation has been associated with this confrontational way of working. This is counterproductive. Orientating information can be presented and offered to a person in a matter-of-fact way so that it can then be accepted or rejected and used in whatever manner that person chooses. Using the approach in this way allows the individual to dictate his or her own care to some extent, and demonstrates a respect for their personhood and sense of agency or control over their lives. The two examples below illustrate the differences in approaches:

1 'Tom, where are you going? It's lunchtime and you need to be in the other direction. Have you forgotten where the dining-room is? Let me take you.'
2 'I'm just going to the dining-room for my lunch. I think it's beef stew today. Would you like to walk along with me?'

In the first example, the worker emphasises the losses Tom is experiencing, presents facts to him without opportunity for him to disagree and takes control from him. This may not only be upsetting but may provoke a degree of anger and distress in Tom. In the second example, however, the worker simply presents information in an everyday manner and presents opportunities for Tom to join in if he so wishes. This approach is less likely to cause problems, and affirms Tom as a valuable human being. It may also help orientate him to his surroundings and environment. By developing this style of working and interacting, workers may reduce the incidence of challenging behaviour with very little effort.

A behavioural approach

As we have already mentioned, most incidents can be predicted and have clearly recognisable patterns to their development. The behavioural approach seeks to form an understanding over time of how the challenging behaviour develops and what it is seeking to communicate so as to increase possibilities for the individual to communicate in the most socially appropriate and acceptable way with the least disruption and distress. Conceptually and in intent, it is therefore a highly ethical approach (Parker, 1993).

The particular model of learning theory which is of use here is operant or instrumental conditioning. As we have already seen, this model proposes that people learn to behave the way they do because of the consequences or rewards received for acting in that particular manner, rather than responding to certain situations in a certain given way. Of course, in practice, the way we think about situations and events, our past experiences, reflection on the behaviour of others and the situation or antecedent event itself may all affect the way we behave. However, we can usefully employ operant theory to reduce behaviour we find challenging and to increase behaviour we find more constructive and more socially and contextually appropriate.

In order to begin a behavioural programme to manage challenging behaviour effectively, a period of observation, monitoring and recording is first necessary. It is important to gain an understanding of the pattern involved: what happens, at what times, in what situations, with whom, and what consequences result from the behaviour – what happens after its occurrence?

Once an hypothesis has been made, it is possible to attempt to find ways in which the challenging behaviour can be decreased and replaced by more acceptable behaviour. To do this, it is necessary to change the consequences that appear to maintain the behaviour, although attention can also be paid to the situation in which it occurs. The situation itself may not lead to the expression of the behaviour, but may indeed be a prompt to suggest to a person to act in a certain way to receive a desired consequence.

Whilst an approach based on these principles can be extremely effective, ethical care needs to be taken. If all staff are not committed to a consistent and thorough approach without wavering then it is most unlikely that benefits will be seen. Also, one criticism levelled against behavioural approaches is that they are very time-consuming and slow. This can be the case, but by investing time and effort in promoting change and encouraging as much independence as possible, it may be that time is saved in the long run. It must be remembered that the challenging behaviour itself can be demanding on time and resources, and any attempt at change may be cost-effective. Behavioural approaches may not be a panacea, but they do offer much in the management of challenging behaviour.

CASE STUDY 7.3: BILL AND VIOLET

Social services had been called because of the incident in which Bill hit Violet. This caused great concern and provided the initial focus of the assessment. At this assessment, however, it became apparent that the main difficulties were, for Violet, Bill's mood swings, aggressive outbursts in general and his talking about his first wife, and for Bill, his frustration and increasing confusion and fear. The initial work, after securing practical support and help for the physical care of Bill, was to monitor the situation surrounding his mood swings and confusion, and to search for patterns. It was also extremely important to pay attention to the sensitive introduction of home care support, and to work with Bill and Violet on this. A hasty introduction, would no doubt have exacerbated the distress, and could have led to more aggressive outbursts, so everything was clearly explained before anything was done. Violet knew that should Bill refuse assistance, this would not be pursued. To help with this, she was provided with a contact to talk through her frustrations and worries, and to help her understand what had happened to Bill, the effects of this, and what might happen in the future.

The pattern emerging from the assessment indicated that it was mornings and early evenings when he became most confused. It was at these times that he retreated into the past and sought his first wife or his friends. If he was confronted or corrected, his distress increased and he became upset and cried, or became aggressive. Having someone with him who talked through his past, asked him about matters of concern, showed him aspects of his life from scrapbooks and photograph albums, and did so in a non-threatening and calm manner, seemed to help him become more relaxed and more content with the world.

A programme designed to help Violet deal with his challenging behaviour and to give him a voice and sense of identity was put into operation after discussion with them both. The programme offered practical help and support. This was something that Bill appreciated. He wanted other company, and responded well to the introduction of a male home care assistant. This led to a request for a place at the local day centre, at which Bill was able to join with other men of his own age and speak about his memories of the war and of boxing. He wanted such an opportunity for social activities, but did not know how to ask. This provided Violet with free time for herself on two days each week.

In order to ensure that both the day centre and the home were as familiar as possible, and to offset distress and frustration at the times he became confused, the social worker, Violet and Bill drew up a list of important features of the home and his life, important events, people and times. A collection of photographs, ornaments and trophies was placed around the house, and a 'map' and routine book was produced by Bill concerning the day centre. This gave him a sense of control and ownership, and demonstrated his sense of humour by his inclusion of little quips about his forgetfulness in the book.

Violet was helped to identify the ways she approached or responded to Bill when he was confused or aggressive, and what possible consequences this elicited. She was then helped to identify other ways of responding, and encouraged to talk more with him, to use a range of calming techniques based on voice control, listening and interest.

This combination of approaches ensured that Violet felt more at ease and in control of her situation, that Bill achieved a greater degree of social contact and stimulation, and that frustration was decreased. Of course, there was a continuing need for social services support and there were difficult times, but for a period of almost eighteen months Bill's challenging behaviour was felt to be manageable by Violet, and both she and Bill stated their appreciation of the change in their relationship.

Activity 7.2

What are the strengths and limitations of the three approaches described above in dealing with challenging behaviours in people with dementia?

Comments

No single approach on its own takes precedence over the others. It is important to refocus on the individual and understand the world, as far as we can, from his or her perspective. The interpersonal skills approach can be very useful in demonstrating concern and value, but can also focus on an individual when the triggers for the challenging behaviour are located elsewhere, perhaps in the care regime and practice itself. The environmental approach reflects a concern for people as being unique, with their own personal biographies, likes and dislikes. It can be expensive to achieve, and with existing resources and time constraints it may not always be considered a priority. The behavioural approach is extremely effective, but again, may mask wider issues and concerns.

The approaches discussed do not offer solutions for dealing with emergency situations. Other policies are needed to detail what can and should be done in such circumstances.

Summary

The concept of 'challenging behaviour' is extremely useful in displacing attention from the *problem* to the underlying *message*: what is the person trying to communicate? Understood in this way, the challenge becomes to discover and respond to the message conveyed by the behaviour, rather than the behaviour itself. There are many ways of attempting to deal with challenging behaviour and to decipher it:

- the sensitive use of interpersonal skills, demonstrating interest in and attention to the person
- a concern for the individuality and life experience of the person by arranging an environment that reflects their needs and provides a flexible but consistent routine
- offering new and adaptive ways in which to express oneself.

These all may diminish potential risk situations for the individual with dementia and staff working with them, and uphold the value, worth and dignity of that person.

8 Counselling and psychotherapy

Introduction

It is not only the person with dementia who can benefit from counselling. Carers experience a range of feelings, emotions and changes to their life-styles. Allowing these to be expressed in an open and non-judgemental relationship can be instrumental in assisting the development of coping strategies. This chapter will introduce some of the ways in which active listening and counselling skills can be used where dementia is an issue. It will not deal with complex psychotherapeutic issues which are beyond the scope of this book and require specialised training, support and super-vision. However, it will describe and promote the use of validation work as a strategy designed to enhance the dignity and quality of life of the person with dementia.

CASE STUDY 8.1: ALFRED AND GLORIA
Alfred and Gloria Whitton had been married for 55 years. They met at the outbreak of World War Two, and married soon after while Alfred was on leave from the army. Throughout their lives they were a very close couple. Since the war ended they had never had a day apart, except for a brief period in hospital for Gloria after the birth of their second child. They worked together in Alfred's greengrocer's shop, enjoying baking, garden-ing and ballroom dancing. Their son and daughter described them as being 'too close'.

After a short illness four years ago, Gloria became tearful, depressed and forgetful. She was unable to continue with her past enjoyments, and Alfred stopped too. According to Alfred, she got no better, in fact she seemed to get worse. He was very worried, and wondered how he would be able to 'recover the real Gloria'.

Gloria herself was aware of great changes to her life, in her memory and functioning. She was increasingly tearful. She often said, 'I don't know what I should do', and asked, 'What is happening to me?'

Model and approach

Put simply, counselling is 'an approach to human communication' (Scrutton, 1989, p. 6). It concerns a process designed to promote understanding and create the conditions in which individuals can make changes for themselves. The term 'psychotherapy' is used in a non-technical sense in this chapter. It refers to a process by which the person's emotional well-being is increased and enhanced. Given their common goals, 'counselling' and 'psychotherapy' will be used interchangeably.

In a recent collection of research papers on counselling and psychotherapy (Dryden, 1996), older people are not mentioned as a specific group of service users – this may be taken as either a good or a bad sign. It may be that the lack of differentiation is meant to be inclusive, giving older people the same opportunities for counselling as younger adults. Unfortunately, this is probably not the case. It is more likely to reflect the general position highlighted by Scrutton (1989) that assumes older people do not need, counselling or cannot usefully engage in it (see also Bytheway, 1994). This view is exacerbated when dementia further 'disables' the potential counsellee. Despite the negative attitudes towards counselling for older people – attitudes often shared by older people themselves – there is a need for counselling among older people with dementia and those caring for them, and value in offering it. By providing the time and space to listen and to explore painful issues in a safe environment, a sense of worth and value can be re-established. It can also help to promote change and strengthen committed relationships, thus allowing caregiving to continue for as long as possible (see Box 8.1).

Scrutton (1989) placed the need for counselling and its potential benefits for older people firmly at centre stage. He indicated that people with dementia could also benefit from these approaches. In fact, his book provided a useful step on the way to the 'new culture of dementia care' (Kitwood and Benson, 1995), emphasising the uniqueness of people in terms of their response to their illness, their life history and their contemporary needs. It set the person in context. Much of Scrutton's work concerns the application of skilled listening and the use of techniques such as reminiscence and life review discussed in other chapters in this book. The message put forward is that communication is not only possible but is essential in working with older people in a validating and dignifying manner.

<table>
<tr><td colspan="2">Box 8.1   The negative and positive value of counselling</td></tr>
<tr><td>Negative views of counselling from</td><td>Positive value of counselling</td></tr>
<tr><td>general public
carers
older people
professionals</td><td>change
re-establish value and worth
preserve identity
preserve caregiving relationships
reduce ill-effects of caring
cost-effective</td></tr>
</table>

The increased recognition of the value of counselling and psychotherapy for people with dementia is clear. Goldsmith (1996, 1997) reiterates forcefully the message that people with dementia are able to communicate and express feelings to a much greater degree than previously thought possible. This, he says, stresses the importance of providing counselling and psychotherapeutic support (Sinason, 1992; Yale, 1996). Giving the individual with dementia opportunities to tell stories allows them to make sense out of their world and lessens suffering (Sutton and Cheston, 1997). Telling stories – the basis of the counselling and psychotherapeutic relationship – is an essential part of the process.

The new culture emphasises the strengths of individuals, and views actions as attempts to communicate (Kitwood and Benson, 1995). Caring is therefore associated with the maintenance and enhancement of personhood. The awareness of individuals with dementia, their uniqueness and the potential for constructive and sensitive communication are highlighted (Froggatt, 1988), and as a consequence, the importance of active listening skills and counselling techniques is promoted (Frank, 1995; Woods, 1995). Carers can also benefit from the application of these skills. It will be useful to review at this point what is involved in these skills and techniques (see Box 8.2).

Box 8.2 The basic features of helping relationships

The basic qualities of helping relationships are well known. Rogers (1951, 1961) described three basic qualities:

- empathy
- warmth
- genuineness.

These core qualities are appreciated by clients and responded to favourably (Hudson and MacDonald, 1986). Carkhuff (1987) adds three more essential conditions to the helping relationship:

- concreteness
- immediacy
- confrontation.

Empathy is the ability to experience the world of another person as if it were one's own. Being empathetic involves being sensitive to the changing experience of the person. It is about understanding and sharing, not judging nor supporting. This is difficult to achieve (Murgatroyd, 1985). It is important to *reflect the content of* what is said – this will help you check that you have understood what is said to you by another person. It is also important to *reflect feelings* – the aim here is to check that underlying and often implicit emotions are also understood. At this point you can also check the congruence of the person's feelings and speech.

In order to achieve *warmth*, the practitioner must respect people as unique individuals and create a safe and trusting environment. By communicating warmth and acceptance to the person who comes for help, one accepts that person regardless of what they say or have done. This is a very difficult frame of mind to develop, but it creates a climate in which the person may feel accepted and in a position to change.

Genuineness relates to a directness and openness in the practitioner's communication. The practitioner has no hidden agenda, concealed thoughts or pretence, but encourages direct and open communication.

To achieve *concreteness*, the practitioner ensures that the person they are helping is specific about the particular meanings they attach to their ideas, images, thoughts, feelings and descriptions. This adds clarity to the communication and helps the practitioner to check their understanding of the person in need.

It is important not to spend too much time talking about the past and past behaviours. The practitioner encourages focus on the immediate and central problem or issue of concern. *Immediacy* can be achieved by asking the person to share their experiences of being with you in the helping relationship as it is happening. This also conveys a sense of value and worth which may be all-important for the person with dementia.

Confrontation does not imply aggression on the part of the practitioner, but refers to pointing out discrepancies and evidence of incongruence between the helper's view and the person in need. Common discrepancies include differences between the real and ideal view of the self, differences between the person's thinking and feelings and what they actually do in practice, and differences between the real world as seen by the practitioner and the fantasy world as seen by the person in need. The skills of effective challenging are contained in Box 8.3.

Box 8.3   The skills of effective challenging (Egan, 1990)

- challenging the client to participate fully in the helping process
- assisting clients to identify blind spots in behaviour and thinking, and assisting in the development of alternatives
- challenging clients to own their problems, to recognise and identify their strengths and potential
- assisting clients to restate the problem in terms of potential solutions
- actively challenging distortions and excuses for inaction
- assisting clients to become aware of the consequences of their behaviours
- assisting client movement from inertia to action.

Greater clarity in thinking may be achieved by using prompts (see Box 8.4).

Box 8.4   Using prompts

Prompts and probes refer to verbal strategies that assist clients to talk about themselves and define issues and problems with greater clarity and specificity. These may include:

- questions
- statements
- interjections.

Questions should serve a specific purpose, be open-ended with the aim of encouraging client talk about specific experiences, behaviours and feelings. *Statements* are indirect requests for more elaboration, whilst an *interjected* word or phrase can assist the process of focusing attention on the subject. These can be responses such as 'Mmm', 'Yes' 'Aha', or even nods. The purpose is to prompt the client to explore the problem situation in greater detail.

Activity 8.1

List the key components of counselling and helping relationships.

Think of reasons why counselling might be helpful for people with dementia.

Comments

We have reviewed six key characteristics for counselling and helping relationships: empathy, genuineness, warmth, being clear, keeping to the present and confronting. These are global characteristics and hold good for all people.

Counselling for people with dementia is often a forgotten area. Social workers see the dementia and the deficits, rather than the person in need behind these. The establishment of a counselling relationship helps people to explore needs and concerns and to communicate fears, hopes and frustrations. The relationship emphasises the uniqueness of the person and their worth as a human being.

CASE STUDY 8.2: ALFRED AND GLORIA

Social services were called by Alfred's and Gloria's daughter to offer practical support with caring. This was achieved by introducing a home help, who also acted as a 'friend and confidante'. The social worker overseeing the case, Ian, felt more was needed. He explored this with both Alfred and Gloria. It was decided that Alfred would meet with Ian for a series of eight sessions to explore his feelings, losses and the future. Gloria was also offered support. A female social worker, Jean, was asked to form a relationship with her and plan towards encouraging her to use her strengths and meet her needs. This involved counselling skills and knowledge.

Alfred was a proud man, nervous of accepting help. Ian tried to put him at his ease by asking him what he wanted to use the time for, and by explaining that nothing was expected of him. Ian reflected back the nervousness and reticence, saying: 'You say you don't really know why you're seeing me. I get the feeling you're a little uncomfortable and on edge.' Alfred agreed and said exactly how he felt. He also felt he had been understood. This short exchange helped Ian to build a rapport with him.

One of Alfred's main worries was that he would be considered 'silly' or 'incapable'. Ian helped him to examine what he meant, and did so in a way that showed acceptance of who he was, what he was doing and the position in which he now found himself. The way Ian sat, looked at Alfred and responded to him helped Alfred to relax and feel that he was being taken seriously.

As the relationship developed and Alfred began to trust the social worker, he was able to respond to the worker's requests for information relating to his thoughts and feelings about Gloria and their present situation. Alfred was helped to see that his protestations of being able to manage without support did not match his feelings of stress. He described Gloria's insistence on following him around the house, continuously asking what he was doing, and his feelings that she was 'looking over his shoulder' all the time. The way he described and expressed this did not meet with his claim to be able to manage. When this was shared with him he was able to see his predicament more clearly. Alfred went on to discuss his need for personal space and time for himself. He said he had always wanted this, but did not know how to say this to Gloria. He also wanted to enjoy past shared interests with Gloria. These thoughts gave him the basis for a plan to work towards.

Scrutton (1989) lists a number of agendas common to the counselling experience in old age. These concern loss of role, functions, significant people and the assumption of a variety of social and cultural stereotypes of ageing. Where dementia is concerned, the sense of loss may be exacerbated on either side: a loss of ability to co-ordinate and perform in expected ways, or the loss of freedom to enjoy retirement for many partners and carers. Whilst it is important to bear in mind these possible agendas, it is also important not to situate the need for counselling purely in the realm of loss. This could lead to minimising or ignoring other needs.

The importance of counselling for people with dementia lies in their awareness, insight and understanding. How frequently has it been said, 'I just don't know what's wrong with me,' or how often have the distress and tears caused by disorientation and confusion been witnessed? Many health and social care practitioners know well, from experience and anecdote, that individuals will respond favourably when listened to, when given the time and space to express their fears and concerns, and when treated as an individual.

One extremely important communication method akin to active listening and psychotherapy, as defined earlier, has been developed by Naomi Feil: validation therapy (Feil, 1992, 1993). Although as a therapy its application is a highly skilled operation and takes specialised training, its principles and strategies may be used to enhance the personhood of those with whom professionals work. The process and understanding can be incorporated easily into our daily practice and approach. It is to this method we now turn.

Validation therapy and validation work

Validation therapy (also known as tuning-in therapy or validation-fantasy therapy) was created in the early 1960s by the American social worker and actress, Naomi Feil. She believed there had been an overreliance on reality orientation, which she thought was confrontational and misplaced (see Chapter 7 on challenging behaviours). She based her approach on person-centred and humanistic philosophies promoted by Rogers in his non-directive approach to therapy. There is an emphasis on respect and a valuing of the uniqueness of persons, their perspectives and world-views (Bleathman and Morton, 1988).

In validation theory it is assumed that the confused person's thoughts and feelings relate to an inner reality or coping strategy designed to help the individual interact with the world around them. The social care practitioner does not actively interpret or analyse, but there is an assumption of meaning behind the words and behaviours. The return to the past is considered to be purposeful in seeking to resolve unfinished conflicts. Validation work or therapy validates these feelings and returns to the past pleasures and pains expressed.

The social worker listens to the person and accepts where they are, encouraging communication and believing the person is struggling to resolve past conflicts. The essence of the work is to encourage and enable the person to express feelings, seeking to validate the rights of people to fantasise, to use private language, and seeking to restore an integrity to the person by allowing them to live through the past when the present no longer holds meaning. The practitioner's role is to act as a link between past associations and present reality.

The process is also based on a stage model of dementia. This is by no means accepted in all circles (see, for instance, the debate in Chapter 1). What is important with validation work is that it is said to be useful for use with people in the later stages or with an advanced dementia (De Klerk Rubin, 1994). It links with reminiscence and life review in its promotion of a constant identity-forming process. The main goals of validation work are:

- to restore a feeling of self-worth
- to reduce stress
- to justify living
- to work towards conflict resolution
- to increase verbal and non-verbal communication
- to improve gait and psychological well-being
- to prevent inward withdrawal
- to reduce the need for chemical and physical restraints.

The skills needed by the practitioner are similar to those employed throughout counselling. Empathy, reflection, creating dialogue and demonstrating an interest are important skills for the social work practitioner to foster.

Many carers have pointed out that they use these skills already. Also, the concern with therapy and the resolution of unfinished business detracts from its potential as a positive framework from which to approach the person with dementia. Not all people who are confused or need their worth validating as an individual do so because of a prior need to relive and assuage their guilt about the past. The approach has been charged with collusion with false realities, but we must remember that everyone constructs their own personal and social worlds on the basis of experience and interaction, and memories are not objective chronologies of events but are charged with emotion and feeling, and are constantly reinterpreted. The approach validates the person and their value and worth where they are, not in terms of the practitioner's perceived reality.

CASE STUDY 8.3: ALFRED AND GLORIA

Gloria had become increasingly confused and distressed. She followed Alfred around the house afraid of being alone, and sobbed uncontrollably not knowing where she was, what was wrong with her and why she was feeling so upset. Jean allowed her to express the pain, confusion and distress and did not try to contradict or dismiss it. It was very real to Gloria. Jean asked her about her fears of being alone, what it was that made her afraid. One memory that came to the fore stemmed from wartime, when she had been informed that Alfred was 'missing in action'. She was frightened that he would disappear, and he was her one constant.

It was not so much this memory that was most valuable about Jean's approach. The fact that she took time to listen, to sit and allow Gloria to cry, to talk about anything that came to mind and to stay with her when she became distressed affirmed Gloria's worth as a person. Whilst there was no set agenda or format to the work with Gloria, she did become more sure of herself and, according to Alfred, seemed to have 'a twinkle in her eye again'.

Activity 8.2

What are the values underpinning the validation approach to work with people with dementia?

Comments

We have noted above that there is an emphasis on respect for persons and their uniqueness. The approach does not seek to privilege one way of looking at the world or reality, but accepts the value of the individuals' perspectives. Validation work is in tune with the new culture of dementia care. It offers the same value to the person with dementia and his or her understanding, worries and wishes as it does to those of others.

Listening skills for practice

The specific technique used by practitioners is not as important as the skills which are used in all approaches, whatever their theoretical base. This is also the case when working with people with dementia. The two main skills are:

- attending or actively being with clients

- active listening.

A person's presence at an important point in another person's life can make a difference. Effective attending tells clients that you are there and are prepared to listen. Egan (1990) distinguishes three levels of attending to clients :

1   microskills.
2   body language.
3   presence.

Microskills relate to how one sits with a client, how interest is conveyed by posture, eye contact and a natural, relaxed manner. However, it is important not to apply too rigid an approach, because of cultural and individual diversity. Social workers need to demonstrate an awareness of their own bodies as a channel for communication. Cues and messages are constantly being sent through our bodies as we interact with clients. The sum of your verbal and non-verbal behaviour should indicate clearly a willingness to work with the client: a commitment to their welfare.

Listening is far more than a simple ability to repeat what has been heard, as we have seen in Chapter 7. It demands a psychological, social and emotional presence with the client. Listening involves four things:

- observing and reading the client's non-verbal behaviour
- listening to and understanding the client's verbal messages
- listening to the person in the context of social settings of their life
- tough-minded listening.

It is often the case that facial expression, bodily motion, voice quality and physiological response convey and communicate far more than the content of clients' words. When working with people with expressive or comprehensive communication difficulties, it is imperative for practitioners to learn how to listen to and read:

- bodily behaviour
- facial expressions
- voice-related behaviour
- observable autonomic physiological responses – these may include quickened breathing, development of rash, blushing, paleness, pupil dilation
- physical characteristics
- general appearance.

These skills assist in validating the worth of a person whose communications are confused and garbled. Non-verbal behaviour can also act as punctuation in the interpersonal situation. It may confirm or repeat what is being said verbally, or it may deny or confuse what is being said verbally. Non-verbal behaviour can strengthen and emphasise the verbal content of the interaction with the client. This may be especially important when working with a carer.

It must also be remembered that the context in which a client lives influences the way people interpret and respond to their lives, so it is important for the practitioner to consider closely the social and cultural background of the person with whom they are working. Tough-minded listening includes identification of the gaps, distortions and dissonance that are part of the client's experience and often-expressed views of reality.

Activity 8.3

List some of the important skills needed in establishing a counselling relationship with a person with dementia. Why are they useful?

Comments

It must be remembered that social workers are not necessarily counsellors, although all social workers use counselling skills in their work. It is important to be aware of how we listen, how we use our bodies, speech and our general manner with people. When working with a person with dementia, it may be that communication is impaired and that we need to listen more intently or need to reflect more to ensure accuracy.

By showing a degree of interest and listening in a way that demonstrates concern, the social worker may convey a message that raises self-esteem and encourages further communication with a trusted person. It also displays the concern and respect we would no doubt demand for our relatives and ourselves.

Summary

This chapter has reviewed the main characteristics of the helping relationship and some of the general features and skills involved in those relationships. These apply to all people, whether young or old. However, attention must be paid to the developmental level and ability of the person involved. When working with people with dementia and their carers, context is all-important and will help practitioners to apply their skills in the most appropriate and effective way.

9 Reminiscence and life review

Introduction

Reminiscence work, reminiscence therapy, life-story work and life review refer to similar but distinct ways of working using an individual's personal biography and life experience. Goldsmith (1996) uses the term 'life story' to refer to the production of a tangible outcome such as a book or video recording (Hargrave, 1994), 'life review' for something less formal, and 'reminiscence' to refer to shared group memories. Murphy and Moyes (1997), on the other hand, see life-story work as a process owned by the individual that can be important at times of change, for celebrating and working through the past, which need not result in the production of a 'book'. In this chapter we will use the term 'reminiscence' to refer broadly to a group or individual activity in which memories are shared with a social worker (Gibson, 1994a), and 'life review' to refer to a more formal process of exploring one's life and identity. Neither need be chronological. We will not examine the therapeutic role of reminiscence and life review since this refers to a more highly-skilled and focused application. Having said this, however, it is noted that therapeutic benefits will often result from the work. The distinction emphasises the general usefulness of reminiscence in increasing enjoyment and social activity. In this chapter we will explore reminiscence work, its development, uses, and how it may be applied for people with dementia.

CASE STUDY 9.1: RESIDENTIAL CARE HOME
A number of residents in a local authority residential care home appeared to staff to be becoming increasingly withdrawn, keeping to themselves and

not talking with other residents. Other residents were overheard making negative comments about these people and saying they were 'odd'. The residents said to be withdrawn all had some degree of memory impairment. Staff became concerned about this and discussed ways of changing this situation between themselves, with workers from outside the unit and the residents themselves. They agreed to allocate special time to each individual, using the unit's keyworker system.

The model and approach

Reminiscence is something we all do (Gillies and James, 1994). It is about telling stories about the past, personal history and individual perceptions of world events. It can be pleasurable, cathartic or therapeutic. It can be spontaneous, or organised and systematic. The skills needed are those important to any interpersonal human activity (Gibson, 1994a). They include:

- active listening
- empathy
- attending to the person
- sensitivity
- respect.

These have been covered in Chapter 8. It is important also to note the value base that is integral to reminiscence work. It values the history, identity and uniqueness of the person. It honours people as social and interactive beings with a great deal to offer and share as a result of their individual life experiences. In these ways it accords well with the emphasis on personhood and professional values.

In the past, oral history was respected as a way of transferring and preserving knowledge and beliefs about the past (Gibson, 1994a). Until recently, however, reminiscence was frowned upon in professional circles, even to the extent that people were discouraged from reminiscing or thought to be abnormal for engaging in it (Dobroff, 1984).

It is generally assumed that the value of reminiscence work was first recognised in the early 1960s by a psychiatrist in New York (Butler, 1963), but its positive and beneficial nature was accepted before this date. The psychologist G. Stanley Hall (1922) reported its value, importance and, indeed, necessity in his work. It is now seen as a 'normal' part of the life review process (Harris, 1988). Coleman (1994) sets this change in acceptance in the context of other social changes in the way old age was approached, the development and rejection of disengagement theory and the rise in developmental psychology. He believes that reminiscence and life review have an evolutionary and protective function for society in passing on self-preservatory knowledge, as well as being good for an individual's emotional and psychological health.

How is it used?

Life review is generally assumed to reflect a more systematic and therapeutic approach to reminiscence. The uses reported are generally therapeutic. Life review has been used in treating older women survivors of childhood sexual abuse (McInnis-Dittrich, 1996), where the choice to participate or not is stressed. It has been used to lessen disorientation and to increase social interaction among older people in care (Tabourne, 1995a, 1995b), especially with those who are depressed (Tabourne, 1995b; Arean et al., 1993). Other therapeutic benefits have been observed, such as increasing self-acceptance (Magee, 1994), promoting a holistic approach to care (Penn, 1994) and as a counselling tool (Webster and Young, 1988; Malde, 1988). Life review has also proven useful in working with gay and lesbian older people (Galassi, 1991).

Reminiscence is also associated with therapy and change, but can be seen as a social and enjoyable activity without being construed as anything more. Therapeutic applications are evident in its use with people who are depressed (Bachar et al., 1991), in raising self-esteem (McGowan, 1994), in reconstructing the identities of older people (Buchanan and Middleton, 1995; Sherman and Peak, 1991) and in stress management for people awaiting surgery (Rybarczyk and Auerbach, 1990) or those in intensive care (Jones, 1995b).

Reminiscence is well documented for use with older people in care settings (Snell, 1991), psychiatric hospitals (Gwyther et al., 1990) and nursing homes (Taft and Nehrke, 1990; Brody, 1990; Rattenbury and Stones, 1989; Orton et al., 1989). It is also well documented for use with people with dementia (Gibson, 1994a; Namazi and Haynes, 1994; Ott, 1993; Martin, 1989). There is still a lack of integrated use in community care, however, because of a continued questioning of its value (George, 1995), and scientific evidence of its benefits remains equivocal (Gillies and James, 1994).

Gibson (1994b) has developed a useful taxonomy from her work with people with dementia which emphasises the diversity of approaches used (see Figure 9.1). These include working with individuals or groups, and being general or specific in theme and topic. Her findings reflect wider research. Large-group, general reminiscence was found to have quite a limited role as an entertainment or diversion. The main gains for people with dementia came from well-planned, well-structured and specific-topic reminiscence and life history, usually in a highly focused, one-to-one situation. This has also been reflected in the authors' own work in the field of

Individual unstructured approach | Individual structured approach

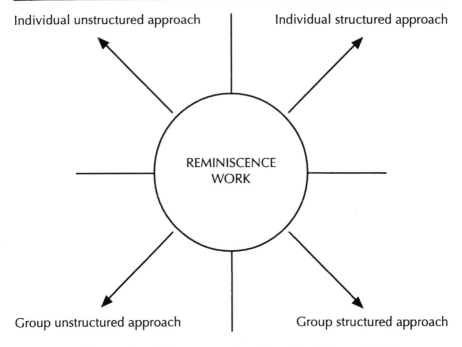

REMINISCENCE
WORK

Group unstructured approach | Group structured approach

Figure 9.1   Types of reminiscence work reviewed in Gibson (1994b)

reminiscence. One particular group co-facilitated by student social workers
rapidly came to the conclusion that one-to-one work would pay greater
dividends. Whilst this may take something away from the social benefits of
joining in small groups, there is still an emphasis on interaction and communication between the participant and facilitator. Also, many of the dis-
tractions found in groups are not present in individually focused sessions.

Reminiscence work is useful in a number of ways. These include:

- dealing with unresolved conflicts
- maintaining self-esteem, identity and feelings of belonging
- forging a continuity with the past
- story-telling and passing on traditions
- enjoying and forming relationships
- reframing the past and planning for the future (Bromley, 1990;
  Coleman, 1987; Goldsmith, 1996).

People with dementia can benefit from reminiscence in grounding their
present relationships and maintaining warm, caring relationships which
may ward off a frightening retreat into isolation and withdrawal (Gibson,
1997). It may also lead to:

- increased participation
- increased spontaneity
- greater socialisation, possibilities for communication and self-expression
- higher self-esteem
- behavioural improvements, and a reduction in the distance between staff and older people (Gibson, 1994a).

There is room for great creativity in planning and designing reminiscence work. In fact, the process itself can be shared and developed by participants. Goldsmith (1996) points out that the person with dementia has years of life experience that influence their present behaviour, and reminiscence can be instrumental in aiding understanding. The first decision to make is whether to work on a one-to-one basis or in a small group. If using a group, it is important to bear in mind the need for clear planning. Important to any group are matters of:

- membership – open or closed
- size – remembering that only small groups should be used with people with dementia
- duration and number of sessions
- venue
- contents of the sessions
- ways of recording and monitoring sessions (see also Figure 10.2).

If work is to be completed with individuals, it can still take the form of reminiscence, but it can be more general and relaxed, rather than involving a systematic life review. However, the need for planning is equally important.

CASE STUDY 9.2: RESIDENTIAL CARE HOME
The keyworkers in the residential unit decided, in consultation with the people they were seeing, to use reminiscence to try and foster a relationship, stimulate conversation and enjoyment. Because of the nature of the memory loss and desire not to participate in groups, individual sessions were arranged. These were informal sessions, but held on a regular basis to establish a pattern, and to allow conversation and social activity to become more commonplace.

Staff members read the case files and met with relatives and previous carers to find out about background. This was used to plan sessions relating to:

- early childhood and school

- family life
- working life
- relationships, family and children
- interests and hobbies
- significant life events
- retirement.

The topics became interchangeable within sessions and often overlapped. Whilst this was a fairly formal structure, facilitators were keen not to impose a rigid chronological approach. The process differed from group to group.

Activity 9.1

What are the main uses of reminiscence for people with dementia?

Are there times when you think that small groups might be more beneficial than one-to-one work?

Comments

Reminiscence work is generally useful in dealing with unresolved conflicts from the past, maintaining self-esteem, identity and feelings of belonging. It helps the person to forge links with the past. It may also be useful in many societies as a means of passing on traditions. The important features are that it can be enjoyable, help establish social relationships and encourage people to reframe their past and plan their future.

As well as the above potential benefits, people with dementia can benefit from the relationships formed by reminiscence work: maintaining warm, caring relationships may ward off a frightening retreat into isolation and withdrawal. It may also lead to increased participation, spontaneity, increased possibilities for communication and self-expression. Benefits seen have also included a rise in people's self-esteem and a reduction in the distance between staff and older people.

When communication, social activity and enjoyment are the focus of the sessions, it may be possible to achieve this in an informal setting comprising two or three participants. This may provide increased benefits. However, the decision to work in groups or with individuals depends upon clear assessment and planning.

Planning for reminiscence

You can choose to use themes or general discussion. You might like to introduce physical objects connected with past events or tasks, play films and music, or even enact role-plays of street parties. However the process is planned, it is essential that you are sensitive to the needs and concerns of a person's past. You will need to:

1 Establish the need.
2 Work out and state the purpose.
3 Determine technical details.
4 Design your programme.
5 Check your participants.
6 Begin your work.
7 Continue the sessions.
8 End and review.

Establish the need

Ask yourself why you want or intend to use or conduct reminiscence work. Is it to further your own development and learning? Is it because your agency uses reminiscence and you have been asked or are expected to conduct reminiscence sessions? Is it because a need has been established to increase communication, opportunities for social activities or to talk about the past with those with whom you work? These reasons are not mutually exclusive, but it is important to be aware of them. You must establish a need in those participating if the sessions are to have value.

Work out and state the purpose

Once a need has been established, you can work out tentatively what you hope to achieve by reminiscence. You will need to revise and clarify the purpose throughout the planning stages. This needs to be done in participation with those who will be taking part in the work.

Determine technical details

It is especially important when conducting reminiscence work with people with dementia to take account of their needs and strengths when deciding whether to work in small groups or with individuals. You will also need to decide where to conduct sessions, who exactly will be involved, how long each session should last, how many sessions there should be overall, what structure the sessions should follow and how the sessions should be recorded.

Design your programme

Return to the original purpose of the group and the needs of those taking part. This will help you decide on a programme and structure for the sessions. Participation in the planning can help to establish bonds and a positive working relationship beforehand. It also demonstrates a concern for and commitment to the value and worth of those taking part. In addition, you should seek to gain information from as wide a range of people as possible. This might include carers and other professionals who know the person or people involved.

A brief outline of a plan is included in Box 9.1. This formed part of a project using student social workers in delivering reminiscence work to a range of settings for people with dementia. The outline comes from a note sent to facilitators after a meeting to determine the structure and character of the sessions. Box 9.2 provides details of a report relating to this work, how it progressed and was used, and what its effects were.

Box 9.1   Programme plan providing details of work undertaken in a reminiscence project

Meeting notes 17 March 1995

There will be eight sessions held between 10 April and 5 May 1995 at Green Park House. These will be held on a twice-weekly basis. It is important to keep in mind the necessity for sessions to proceed at the pace of the participants and for themes/focus to be flexible to account for their needs.

There will be an introductory session held to gain information about likes and dislikes and to begin to form a working relationship. Following this session, plans can be made to prepare sessions around certain themes of interest. In order to plan effectively and to be prepared, project facilitators will prepare material for two reminiscence sessions each. These include:

- wartime in North Town and wider – Lucy and Martin

- places of interest and where people grew up – Lucy
- fishing, industry and occupations – Martin
- school days – Petra
- fashions – Petra
- films, film stars and music – Jean
- superstitions and games – Jean.

Other topics for sessions may include famous people from North Town, North Town in history, transport in North Town, cinemas and dance halls, holidays, buildings, changes seen in North Town.

Facilitators will prepare brief notes about the important components and features of their topics which may be used by others in the group. They will also seek to make four or more photocopies of pictures that might evoke comment and rememberings. These can be taken from local history resources and booklets, newspapers and other sources. The question of resources is important. If any materials – photographs, newspapers, artifacts, etc. – can be located, please let everyone know. We need to develop a resource 'booklet' for use when planning sessions

It is expected that these topics will provide a focus and key to eliciting reminiscences and will generate information about personal lives and family histories. Whilst some of these memories and rememberings may be tinged with sadness, and need to be so, each session should attempt to end on a positive note. Sessions themselves should be no longer than 40 minutes, perhaps nearer 30 minutes. If people wish to leave during the session – for whatever reasons – this should be respected.

Box 9.2   The results of prior planning

Prior to taking part in the reminiscence groups and individual sessions, facilitators were given selected readings relating to reminiscence work and dementia and attended a short workshop on reminiscence and groupwork skills. They had a regular supervision meeting to report back on progress and any issues arising.

Topics and themes were picked in collaboration with participants, who were asked for likes and interests, staff were asked about particular likes and dislikes, and facilitators undertook research into and collected materials on a range of topics and themes of interest.

Facilitators used a variety of different media to stimulate discussion, interest, and to facilitate enjoyment in the sessions. The media chosen related to different types of sensory stimulation and were taken from a wide range of sources. Media and stimulus material included:

- visual – photographs, slides, videos; books, postcards, news-papers and magazines, toys and games, pets, clothes, kitchen implements, old gramophone, pens and slates
- audio – records, cassette tapes, live music, sound effects
- tactile – pet chinchilla rabbit, pens, shells and sand, books, news-papers, magazines and ration books, toys and games, clothes, essential oils
- olfactory – essential oils
- taste – brandy snaps, rock, tea and biscuits.

Norris (1986) and Gibson (1994a) emphasise the use of as wide a range of materials as possible to stimulate participants in reminiscence. Using different materials means it more likely that as many as possible will be able to participate in the session.

Check your participants

It is important to undertake prior planning before finally determining who wishes to and is able to take part. This will differ according to the purpose and structure of the work. For instance, if the work is to be undertaken with individuals, it may be that a need was first identified for one person. Planning may have been carried out with that individual in mind, and the question of participation may be settled almost prior to making plans. For a small group this may be very different. A general need may be recognised for opportunities for communication, social activity and contact. The final decision concerning participants may not be made until planning has been completed and feasibility checked.

Begin your work

A first introductory session during which plans and arrangements can be introduced, shared and finalised is very important. This can be quite infor-mal and relaxed. It is important to begin in this way even if you know the person/people you will be working with. It makes the work special and something to be noted.

Continue the sessions

Remember to be flexible to the needs of the individual or group and to be sensitive to changes in other aspects of people's lives. This may affect your programme and require you to make changes at the last minute. Be prepared for this. It is always worthwhile planning for contingencies before they occur.

After each session, you should check with participants to see how they felt about the sessions, and with others around the person. Also record your observations.

End and review

It is always important to plan for endings and to ensure that participants are well prepared. You need to introduce the notion of endings from the first session onwards, but also refer to the number of sessions left during each one. This will help offset some of the emotion that can be associated with endings, but may not account for it all nor for the special circumstances that may arise from working with people with dementia. They may not remember your plans. It is therefore useful to end on a positive high note. Plan the final session to be almost like a party or celebration of what you have done in previous weeks.

Providing tea and cakes can give the final session a more relaxed feel. It can help to set the scene for a review of the work and to gain important comments and feedback from participants. Box 9.3 provides part of a report concerning the student social workers and their evaluation. This prompted a review of recording and evaluation procedures for future sessions.

Box 9.3   Evaluating the group

The main methods of evaluation of the group and individual sessions consisted of written reports produced by the facilitators. These included staff and participant comments. At times individual recording sheets were used. Unfortunately, these were not applied in a systematic way. Other feedback was sought from staff and participants, and some sessions have been directly observed.

It is important to record what happened in each group and what responses were made by people participating. Norris (1986), Bender et al. (1987), Webster (1993) and Gibson (1994a) are clear about the need for evaluation, and have developed forms and schedules to assist recording. The important point is to ensure that information is recorded systematically in a way that can be understood easily by another person. The purpose of evaluation and review will influence how and what is recorded, but it is probably best to include the views of participants, other staff caring for participants and the person facilitating the session. Carers may also have helpful comments to add. Evaluation sheets can be as simple as recording the basic details of that group, what happened, what was used and who was there, and the views and observations from all involved. This will help

---

Session evaluation sheet

Name:

Date:

Focus of session:

Views of participant:

    What did you like best about today's session?

    What would you change about today's session?

    Any other comments?

Views of staff:

Worker comments/observations:

Figure 9.2 Evaluation sheet

you to plan future work and to adapt it to the needs of participants. (A sample recording form is given in Figure 9.2).

Activity 9.2

How might you reduce the effect of possible pitfalls in reminiscence work in dementia care?

Comments

Planning and assessment are essential in reminiscence work. Of course, it is not always possible to account for all possible problems, but by planning the technical details they can be minimised. It is also important to get to know the participants beforehand and to ensure that the work is participative and runs at the pace and according to the needs and interests of participants. In this way not only is the work more likely to be successful but it is grounded in the values of respect for the person and an acknowledgement of their potential to interact.

CASE STUDY 9.3: RESIDENTIAL CARE HOME

The sessions went down well overall. The main outcome being that residents became more talkative and keen to join in activities on the unit. For one resident, however, there was no positive change. In fact, he seemed to deteriorate. Recording sheets were used, and these indicated that after each session he became upset, spending more time crying in his room. He hardly spoke to the worker, and added no comments to his view of the sessions. It was felt that reminiscence was not appropriate for this man, and this was respected. The sheet of another person indicated how the majority of sessions proceeded and what their outcome was (see Figure 9.3).

The evaluations of sessions allowed staff to plan with residents for future sessions and work, and to reflect on what worked, when, and to formulate ideas as to why.

Throughout the process it is essential to remember:

- Be flexible
- Be sensitive
- Be creative.

Session evaluation sheet

Name: *Roy Smith*

Date: *23 June*

Focus of session: *School days*

Views of participant:

What did you like best about today's session?
I liked remembering the games we played, the football and thinking of Charles Diamond. It's nice to remember your friends.
What would you change about today's session?
Nothing really, but I'd like to talk again.
Any other comments?
Not really. I enjoyed it. It would be nice if we could meet up with old friends sometime.

Views of staff:
Roy seemed a little withdrawn after today's session but spoke a lot about it in the evening. He talked about sport at school and about his friends. He seemed to have enjoyed himself in the end.

Worker comments/observations:
Roy was reflective today. He had a lot more to say than usual and seemed to wander off to past times with his friends and games. I thought the session went well and it made me remember things I thought I had forgotten.

Figure 9.3   Completed evaluation sheet

It is important to keep in mind that the sessions are for the participants to use however they wish, and that progress must take place at their own pace, not yours. Figure 9.4 provides a visual check to determine the reasons for the reminiscence work. Whilst social workers and their agencies can gain benefit from reminiscence, and personal wishes and agency operations are not necessarily contrary to working on behalf of clients, the sessions

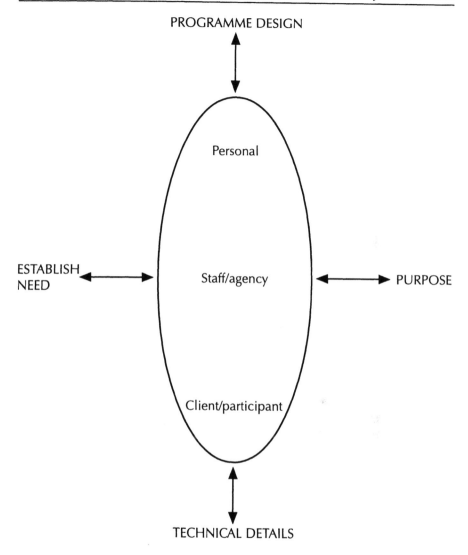

Figure 9.4 Motivations influencing reminiscence work

will be successful, enjoyable and beneficial only if a client need is established. The client must always be the prime consideration in planning, designing and conducting reminiscence work.

Activity 9.3

Begin to plan what themes and interests you intend to prepare for six to eight reminiscence sessions. Consider what resources you might need, what preparation, what possible consequences may arise, and how these will be handled. Write a brief schedule for these sessions.

Comments

To a large extent it will be up to you and the people with whom you are working to determine what form the sessions will take. It is essential that they match the pace of the person involved, pay attention to the needs and topics which they would like to cover, and are flexible enough to respond to quickly changing situations and needs. Plan your session schedule in conjunction with a clear overall plan for your work in dementia care.

Summary

In this chapter we have looked at reminiscence work with people with dementia, why it is useful, and how to begin to prepare for it. It can be a very positive experience for people taking part, but can, of course, often evoke strong and sometimes painful emotions. The social worker must be aware of the need for sensitivity and flexibility in the approach, and must be prepared to change and adapt sessions and to work at the pace of the participant.

The approach is highly ethical if used in these ways. It shows a respect for the history of individuals, and acknowledges that people are social beings and have a need to share, teach and continue to review and experience aspects of their lives.

10 Working in groups

Introduction

Many of the interventions we have discussed so far may be undertaken in group settings as well as individually. However, it is important to consider the use of groups in their own right, since they represent an extremely powerful and effective medium for influencing and directing change. In this chapter we will consider a variety of aspects and characteristics of groups, and their uses for older people with dementia and their carers.

CASE STUDY 10.1: MARY AND THE DAY CENTRE

Each year Highlands Day Centre held a fête to raise funds and to forge links with the surrounding community. Carers of those who attended the day centre often gave things that they had made for sale at the fête. One year, however, a member of the day centre staff thought the sale would provide a useful focus for an activity group for members of the centre to contribute directly to the fête. She identified a number of people who had worked in or enjoyed dress-making throughout their lives. Many of these people had not made anything for a number of years, and other staff and carers were sceptical whether this was a good idea. Mary, the day centre social worker, was not discouraged, and presented an idea to a team meeting based on her discussions with members. It was agreed that she should help establish a group to make something for the fête.

Mary had prior experience in groupwork, and found that people generally encouraged and supported each other. She ran a carer support group for people whose relatives attended the day centre. This was firmly established and recognised as providing useful support and assistance.

Model and approach

When any more than two people join together, a group of some description is formed. This makes it a particularly complex matter to define and determine the various types of groups. Heap (1977) offers a very useful overview of group types for those working in social work and social care situations. He makes an important distinction between *primary* and *secondary* groups. A primary group is one in which numbers are small enough to allow face-to-face contact, the group continues over a certain length of time allowing relationships to develop, and these relationships generate mutual identification and influence. Families, peer groups and residential or day care settings are examples of this type of group. It is these groups which we shall concentrate on throughout this chapter.

A secondary group is a larger affiliation in which relationships are not so close. In fact, they may be based upon a common characteristic or interest. An example of a secondary group may be football team supporters or followers of a particular religion. It may also be the stereotyped group consisting of all people with dementia. As we have noted earlier, attitudes towards individuals are influenced by beliefs about common deficits, behaviours and prognoses. This grouping demonstrates a wider need for societal education and the promotion of personhood in social and healthcare settings. In the services provided, policies devised and in the individual work carried out, social workers can promote the uniqueness and worth of people with dementia.

Sutton (1994) identifies groups by their purpose and suggests there are four basic types:

1 *Therapeutic groups* – in these, the purpose is change and the group is led by professionals, Fatout (1992) describes a range of methods used in these types of groups, including person-centred counselling, behavioural approaches, gestalt therapy, transactional analysis and reality therapy.
2 *Support groups* – these may be formed by social care practitioners in the first instance, but these practitioners become less important to the group and act as facilitators to help participants explore issues or to put them in touch with relevant services.
3 *Self-help groups* – these may develop from support groups and may or may not have a social care practitioner involved at times; the participants come together to work on a shared concern and to offer each other support, help and advice.
4 *Self-directed groups* – in these, participants take charge, set the purpose and direct the group; Mullender and Ward (1991) describe such a group in terms of empowerment.

When working with people with dementia and their carers there are a number of groups in which individuals may participate, and a range of types in which the social care practitioner may be involved (see Box 10.1). These categories are not exhaustive and are not meant to be restrictive. They illustrate the types of group most frequently used at present. Although the boxes 'Self-help group' and 'Self-directed group' are left empty in relation to people with dementia, the social work practitioner can enable and encourage individuals to seek change on their own behalf.

Groups for people with dementia are generally undertaken in day care and residential settings and in statutory, profit making and non profit making agencies. The positive elements of respect for the dignity and value of individuals is emphasised by the increased demand for support groups for people with dementia (Yale, 1996; Keady, 1997). There is also an increase in demand for carer support groups in response to the growing numbers of carers (Benbow, 1997) and a reported use in stress and anger reduction to assist the process of caregiving (Phair, 1997) which may contribute to the prevention of abuse in caregiving relationships (see Chapter 11 and Browne and Herbert, 1997). There is still an element of stigma attached to the offer of attendance at a support group, however. Some carers may see it as a slight on their ability to cope and care (Clarke, 1997), so a sensitive approach needs to be taken. A very practical guide to using groups with older people, including people with dementia, is provided by Bender et al. (1987).

Social workers are involved in working with groups on a number of different levels. First of all, of course, they are usually members of teams, often comprising other disciplines and workers. To work in this kind of environment one needs to develop an understanding of and personal approach to one's work as an individual and how one interacts with others in a manner that facilitates the achievement of team goals and objectives. It is important to the team working with people with dementia to have a clear value base emphasising both rights and responsibilities, that sees the person first and the disability second. Explicit policies and procedures may set out the ground rules, but the new culture of personhood must be internalised to have greatest effect in practice.

What is usually understood by 'working in groups', however, is the social worker leading, facilitating or empowering people in numbers greater than one. A group can comprise members of a family (however this may be understood) who each develop their own patterns and ways of working, their own rules, responsibilities, their own roles and styles of interacting. At this level, it is often true to say that most if not all social workers engage in groupwork when working with people with dementia.

Working with groups of people brought together for a common purpose or reason has developed as a specific form of social work practice, and it is this to which people most commonly refer when discussing social

Box 10.1	Main types of group for people with dementia and their carers			
	Therapeutic groups	Support groups	Self-help groups	Self-directed groups
Person with dementia	• Reminiscence groups • Reality orientation group • Psychotherapeutic group • Healthy living group • Physiotherapy group • Stress management group	• Activity and social group. This may include many of the activities under 'Therapeutic groups' where the emphasis is on social contact and support		
Carer	• Psychotherapeutic group • Stress management group	• Carer support group	• Voluntary self-help groups, such as Alzheimer's Disease Society. They may also develop from carer support groups	• Groups directed at social change on a local or wider level

groupwork. All groups share common characteristics. A basic understanding of these and the processes at work in groups is important for social work practice. It is to these that we now turn.

Groups form and develop over time. The development of groups – how they come into being and progress – is closely related to how the criteria for membership are established, or group composition. Groups may be *compulsory* by virtue of a context such as residential care. The compulsory nature of the group does not rule out common purpose, however. It may be that a number of individuals in residential care have little choice with whom they live, but they may be able to gain a sense of belonging, cohesion, purpose and decisionmaking by pursuing a common interest together. In one situation this was achieved by setting up a music group. One individual played the piano, staff helped by providing cassette tapes and a player, and other residents sang songs or simply enjoyed the music without actively taking part.

Other groups may be referred to as *formed*. This might relate to carer support groups, self-help groups and some reminiscence groups. These are usually initiated by the social work practitioner. The third type can be referred to as a *natural* group that arises spontaneously as a result of circumstances and chance. A shared interest in walking and botany led to the establishment of friendships among members of a carer support group. A walking group developed from this group. It continued beyond the life of the original support group, and offered support to those who joined.

Newly formed groups of all types pass through a number of stages. Tuckman (1965) identified these stages as:

1 forming.
2 storming.
3 norming.
4 performing.

At first there is considerable anxiety about group tasks and focus, and a frantic search for a group leader. This is followed, in the storming phase, by conflict, challenges and the development of sub-groups. The group then consolidates, gains greater stability and develops norms prior to paying increased attention to the task and the solution of issues and concerns in its performing stage.

CASE STUDY 10.2: MARY AND THE DAY CENTRE

There were five women at the day centre who wanted to join Mary's dressmaking group. In the initial stages she met with them to decide exactly what they would do for the fête. The composition of the group was forced, in that members attended the same day centre, but attendance was determined by interest and a wish to do some dress-making. After much deliberation, the group decided to make a set of patchwork cushion covers. Members looked to Mary for a lead and a decision, but at this stage she felt it best to facilitate discussion and to allow everyone involved to contribute ideas and suggestions. This approach gave all five the opportunity to discuss their past experiences, their wants and wishes, to disagree and argue, and to develop a greater understanding of each other.

During the formative stage, when arguments continued, Mary was spoken to by other members in the day centre who felt she was being too ambitious and that the group was causing damage, rather than providing benefits. Mary used her knowledge of group formation to allay their fears, or at least offer an alternative explanation of what was happening.

Having decided on a course of action, the next phase was one of consolidation. Tasks were allotted and agreed. They all joined in choosing the material, but three of the group acted as material cutters to help the others who found using scissors difficult. One of those who could use scissors found she could not sew as well as she could previously. She was paired with another member who could. In all, eight cushions were made for the fête and all of them sold. This achievement was viewed very positively by those involved, and also by staff who at first thought the idea misguided. Mary worked with other day centre staff and members to establish and continue this kind of craft group, linking it with an oral history project on household skills.

Activity 10.1

List some of the types of group and some of the stages through which a group might pass during its course.

What might you need to take into account for people with dementia?

Comments

Groups may be used for therapeutic purposes, supportive reasons and may be 'self-help' or professionally led. However, all groups tend to pass through a number of stages, although in practice these become blurred and the sequence may change. The 'forming, storming, norming and performing' model is useful in giving an idea of the various stages in the life of a group.

Using groupwork for people with dementia may raise some special issues. It may be that stages are not reached, or are reached time and again because participants' memories and orientation is impaired. Much depends on the purpose of the group. Whilst therapeutic groups are not common, they may be used under certain circumstances, especially in the early stages if dementia or after diagnosis. It is more likely that support groups are being considered, and this is where prior planning is important. The special needs of participants must be known and taken into account in the groups.

As well as an understanding of the stages groups pass through, it is useful to have an understanding of some of the common elements and components involved in working with groups. An extremely useful and accessible introduction is provided by Whitaker (1985). She outlines 17 important decisions and tasks to bear in mind when considering setting up and working with groups (see Box 10.2). This is oriented towards practitioner-initiated groups, and mainly for those concerned with helping or therapeutic purposes. However, the considerations outlined are useful for all types of groups.

Box 10.2 Important considerations in setting up a group

- Decide on the group's membership
- Clearly state expected benefits of the group
- Tailor the group to members' needs
- Decide on group leader(s)
- Work out the basic structure and character of the group
- Undertake a cost-benefit analysis
- Make detailed structure and operational policy
- Identify means of evaluation of the group
- Find means of support for facilitators
- Make individual commitment to the group
- Identify group membership and determine the need for preparatory work
- Decide how to begin the group
- Determine the role of facilitator
- Make any final changes necessary to the structure
- Decide how to deal with unexpected consequences during the life of the group
- Decide when and how to end the group
- Decide about future work in the light of experience.

CASE STUDY 10.3: MARY AND THE DAY CENTRE

It is worth spending a little time looking in more detail at Mary's work with this group and the issues she took into consideration to establish it.

As mentioned previously, membership was based primarily on interest rather than skill, since the emphasis was on enjoyment, occupation and activity rather than making perfect items. Because of this and the special needs of some members, arising from arthritis, visual impairment and sequencing difficulties, the plan to make patchwork cushion covers was chosen. Whilst some staff thought there might be problems and participants might feel they had failed by not completing tasks, Mary ensured that people undertook tasks they felt comfortable with, and she constantly emphasised the enjoyment factor rather than production.

The group met twice each week at the day centre. It was facilitated by Mary, but each participant was encouraged to have an equal say in its running. This participation was also evident in the evaluation procedures. Mary herself checked people's attendance, what they said about the tasks and what she observed, whilst participants were themselves encouraged to comment on the usefulness or otherwise of the group.

In this group there was a natural end which helped to focus it. The original motivation for the group consisted of making something for the annual fête. There was a specific date planned ahead for this. However, the group was enjoyed so much by participants and the benefits of increased communication, smiles and reported satisfaction by carers were such that the group continued beyond this time.

Activity 10.2

Read the following case vignette and consider what you might need to take into account.

You have been asked to help a new group of residents set up a support group to help them adjust to life in residential care. The prospective participants are predominantly female, outnumbering the males six to two. They all have dementia and have moved into residential care within the last month.

Comments

First of all it would be important to examine the reasons for the request and what purpose the group would serve for these residents. Having reached agreement or gained a variety of ideas, these could be tested with each prospective participant. In this way you would be able to check who wanted to be involved. Personal biographies, special needs arising from the dementia, from their life history or from the situation in which they now found themselves would need to be examined and accounted for. It may be that a female-only group is possible, or the men perhaps feel uncomfortable.

After prior planning and assessment work you could begin to organise either a programme or a series of more informal meetings to begin the group.

Box 10.3   Group characteristics

- Groups develop particular moods and atmospheres
- Shared themes can develop within groups
- Groups evolve norms and belief systems
- Groups vary in cohesiveness and in the permeability of their boundaries
- Groups develop and change their character over time
- Persons occupy different positions within the group in terms of power, centrality, being liked or disliked which may change throughout the course of the group
- Individuals sometimes find one or two others to whom they are especially close or find particularly important to them
- Social comparison may take place within the group
- Groups provide environments in which members can observe the actions and utterances of others and then observe the consequences of these
- Groups can provide a forum for receiving feedback from others concerning behaviour and participation in the group
- A group may provide the environment in which new behaviours can be tried out
- Members of a group may collide and jostle for comfortable positions, and collude with others to achieve this.

An understanding of these common characteristics helps the social work practitioner to be aware of possible changes and not to overreact to certain group events or situations. If it is in agreement with the predetermined and shared purpose of the group, an understanding of the characteristics can facilitate a smoother achievement of goals.

Of course, the overall purpose of the group must be to maximise potential benefits to group members. There may also be a number of sub-purposes and instrumental purposes that may contribute to the achievement of the overall purpose.

Instrumental purposes increase the safety and functioning of the group by setting out guidance and targets for accomplishment. Further purposes helping towards this include keeping in mind the internal workings of the group during operation, and reflecting on the work out of sessions. Considerable effort in the planning stages will help achieve the purpose, and final assessment and evaluation is integral to effective future planning.

Throughout the stages of a group's life, there are a range of special features and characteristics of groups that it is essential to bear in mind when planning, running, facilitating or assisting in setting them up as a medium to help people (see Box 10.3; Whitaker, 1985).

Activity 10.3

Refer to the group characteristics mentioned above, and think of ways in which they might apply to groupwork for people with dementia.

Comments

Each groupwork situation is different, but many of the characteristics apply whatever the nature, purpose and composition of the group. You may have thought about a group in which one member talked at length about their past and how they did things in their family, often to the consternation of others. The other group members may have dealt with this by ignoring this person's comments or rudely shouting them down, or they may have capitulated to their domination. The repetition of tales and histories and the search for a previously known and non-threatening time may fragment larger groups and create smaller cliques. When working with people with dementia, it is usually best to work only with small groups.

CASE STUDY 10.4: MARY AND THE DAY CENTRE
If Mary had not had an understanding of groupwork she might not have proceeded with the group because of the antipathy of some other staff. However, her understanding also helped her to deal with the development of ideas and some of the arguments and interpersonal clashes that arose

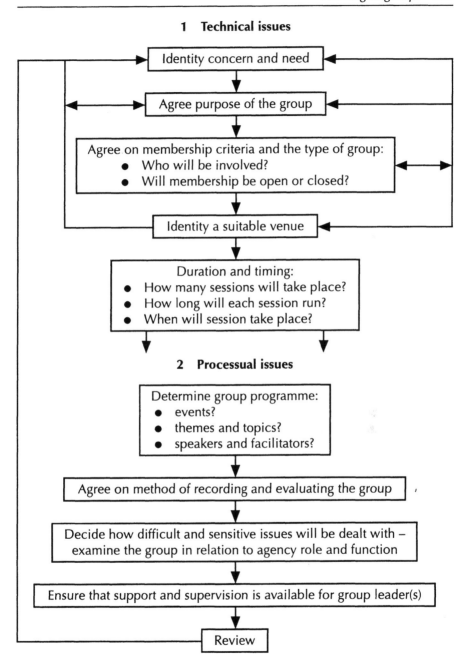

1 Technical issues

Identity concern and need

Agree purpose of the group

Agree on membership criteria and the type of group:
- Who will be involved?
- Will membership be open or closed?

Identity a suitable venue

Duration and timing:
- How many sessions will take place?
- How long will each session run?
- When will session take place?

2 Processual issues

Determine group programme:
- events?
- themes and topics?
- speakers and facilitators?

Agree on method of recording and evaluating the group

Decide how difficult and sensitive issues will be dealt with – examine the group in relation to agency role and function

Ensure that support and supervision is available for group leader(s)

Review

Figure 10.1   Groupwork flowchart

between members. The success of this was, in part, due to Mary taking a facilitator role rather than imposing her view on others. She allowed comparisons to take place, and encouraged help and support for each other to develop.

In some groups this relaxed approach might not have worked and a more directive approach might have been necessary. Mary was aware of this, and ensured she was aware of conflicts and issues which might have become upsetting for some members. It was fortunate that this did not occur in this group.

Social groupwork for people with dementia and their carers is a practical activity aimed at enabling and enhancing skills, functioning and feelings of positive self-worth. The flow-chart in Figure 10.1 provides a summary of the tasks and considerations necessary for effective groupwork. These are applicable whether the group is led or facilitated by a professional or initiated by a group member. In the latter case the social worker may be instrumental in sharing knowledge with group members to increase the potential for effective groupwork.

Group focal conflict theory

An interesting model used to understand the ways some groups proceed, and solve issues has been developed, known as the *group focal conflict model*. It will be useful to look at this model and how it relates to groupwork for people with dementia and their carers.

Whitaker (1985) introduces the concept of *group solution* as a model encompassing many of the group characteristics discussed previously. Norms and belief systems provide a safety function to contain the fears and anxieties of the group within certain limits whilst allowing for further exploration of some of these. By adopting such systems, the group is able to generate its own solution. The concept of group solution is among those encompassed by the model of group functioning known as *group focal conflict theory* (see Figure 10.2). This, in turn, is built upon the theory which explains intrapersonal dynamics as a nuclear focal conflict.

Nuclear (or individual and internal) conflicts are established as a consequence of one's early life experiences. Habitual coping patterns develop. These are resonant with the original conflict, which comprises a core wish set against some associated fear or guilt. The conflict sometimes leads to a solution containing the fears, and sometimes allows for the satisfaction of the wishes.

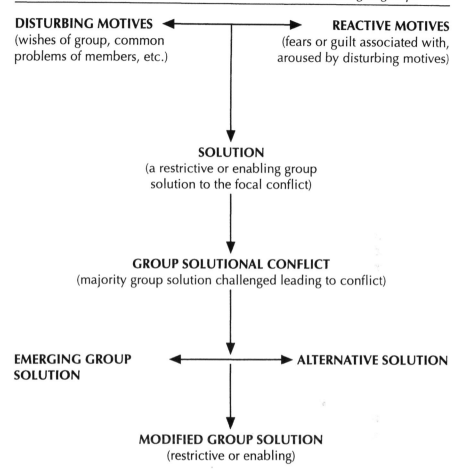

Source: Adapted from Heap (1977).

Figure 10.2 The group focal conflict model

The emergence of a shared wish is often observed in group situations. In terms of group focal conflict theory, this is known as the *disturbing motive*. If nothing prevents the expression of this wish, it can emerge as a theme for group discussion. However, it is often accompanied by a related shared fear or guilt that militates against its expression. This would be called the *reactive motive*. It is these two associated phenomena that constitute the *group focal conflict*.

The group reacts to the focal conflict by seeking a solution. A *restrictive solution* that concentrates on the fears at the expense of the wish and precludes useful problem exploration, although it contains acceptable anxiety, may result. However, an *enabling solution* that allows the expression of the wish, facilitates exploration and allays group fears may result. Sometimes a *solutional conflict* may emerge. This happens when a member of the group challenges an emerging solution and attempts to prevent it being established. If a solutional conflict arises, it needs to be resolved. A further conflict between the unconsolidated group solution and an alternative solution results in a modified group solution.

The group focal conflict model continually evolves throughout each successive phase of group development. At some stages a restrictive solution may be necessary to allay the anxieties of group members. If the group is working well, it should move to more enabling solutions as it becomes established. Also, recurring themes permeate the phases of group life. One topic may be focal at one time, giving way to others, and possibly returning later. The position of an individual in the group may also alter during each particular phase and focal conflict, depending on his or her reaction to it.

Mood, atmosphere and group cohesion may act as restrictive or enabling solutions. If leaders are aware of the focal conflict model, they may have a better understanding of whether or not that particular solution needs influencing. Facilitating the development of more enabling solutions increases opportunities for social comparison, spectatorship, giving and receiving feedback, and testing out new behaviours. The leader can take on a directive role in challenging the development of distorted beliefs and thinking patterns that arise and hamper the progress of the group.

It may also be that an individual who occupies a *deviant* position with respect to an emerging solution is afforded increased opportunities for self-examination and development. Being aware of this allows the leader not to 'rush to save' this member. The model is also useful for designing a group and selecting for it. It can help answer such questions as who is most likely to benefit and under what circumstances.

The model helps the leader focus on when to intervene. In the initial stages a restrictive solution may be necessary to the maintenance of the group, but may at a later stage be dropped and replaced by a more enabling solution. Unless it will be harmful to an individual, it is probably best if the leader does not directly influence a restrictive solution. However, by alleviating fears, the leader can facilitate a move from a restrictive solution.

CASE STUDY 10.5: MARY AND THE CARER SUPPORT GROUP

Mary also ran a carer support group. Reference to this may help to illustrate how the group focal conflict model can be useful in working with carers.

The group had formed as a result of expressed needs by a number of carers of people with dementia. A need for support, information and social contact formed its initial basis. During the group it transpired that members wanted to complain about the stress and demands of caring, and that they wished they did not have to do it. This was countered by feelings of guilt, worry about what other carers might say in and outside the group, and beliefs that they ought to be caring for their relatives. These two positions formed a focus of conflict for the group.

The group went through many developments throughout its life. At first the worries and concerns prevented expression of the strong feelings against caring. The group seemed tense, but complaints were not mentioned explicitly, and when anything negative was said about caring the group quickly moved on to another subject. This formed a restrictive solution that, at that stage in the group's life, was functional and allowed members to bond and become more trusting of one another. Allowing this period of denial paved the way for later exploration of negative feelings when one member of the group spoke about her wedding day and the fact that her mother-in-law, for whom she now cared, took her to one side and informed her she would never be good enough for her son.

Once the group trusted one another and saw each other with faults, positives, similarities and differences, they began to open up, and a long period in one session was devoted to the 'unfairness' of their present position, and their wish that they did not have to care. The group decided that airing grievances was beneficial and that they should continue to do this in the group's safe and supportive environment. Many members expressed relief and a feeling of being able to cope with caring much better after complaining about it in the group.

Not everyone agreed with this solution, however. Two members believed that complaining and speaking about the person they cared for in a negative way was, for them, wrong, and betrayed the needs of those people. This allowed for further discussion about the solution to the group's need. A modified solution was found in which both positive experiences and concerns could be discussed, and whereby no one was pressured to listen to or agree with the statements of others, but neither was anyone to blame or judge other members for their feelings.

This modified group solution allowed the group to continue and to gain from the variety of speakers and learning on offer. It did require a group facilitator who understood basic group processes and who was able to allow matters to develop and to allow conflict and some upset at times.

Summary

This chapter has covered the basic uses of groups in working with people with dementia and their carers. There are, as we have seen, many different types of groups and many reasons for working in groups, not least their cost-efficiency and potential for increasing motivation and social learning. Whatever the purpose of the group, its composition and type, all seem to share certain characteristics and processes and go through a variety of stages through the course of their life. It is therefore important to have an understanding of these in order to be able to work most effectively with the group and its members.

11 Dementia and elder abuse

Introduction

In recent years there has been a gradual increase in concern about the abuse and neglect of elderly people. The predominant focus has been on abuse of elders by their carers in the domestic setting, although increasingly there has been a move towards consideration of abuse occurring within institutional settings (Clough, 1996). Elder abuse is not a new phenomenon (Stearns, 1986), but only since 1988 has the problem begun to be addressed in the United Kingdom.

CASE STUDY 11.1: STANLEY AND GRACE

Stanley White was 77 years old when he was referred to his local social services department by the family GP. He had had a minor stroke some two years previously, and despite having high blood pressure, appeared to have recovered well from it. Recently, however, his wife Grace had noticed some changes in his personality, and his memory appeared to be worse. Stanley was showing swings in mood, was increasingly irritable and had become very verbally aggressive on several occasions as a result of minor disagreements with other members of the family. The situation had come to a head when Stanley had become physically violent towards his wife during an argument with her. His son, Graham, who was present at the time, had intervened in an attempt to protect his mother, and both men and Grace had had to be treated for minor injuries by the locum GP who was called out as it was a weekend. The locum had requested further action within the situation from the family GP.

The GP contacted social services following a discussion with the couple and their family (a son and two daughters). All were expressing concern about Stanley's behaviour and its effects and were asking for assistance with this. They were agreeable to a referral to social services. Grace was upset and somewhat afraid of her husband, commenting that this type of situation had never occurred during their married life; the children echoed the change in Stanley's behaviour from a loving and devoted father to an argumentative tyrant.

The social worker who visited the family held a number of discussions with the whole family as part of the assessment, whilst retaining a clear focus on Stanley and Grace as a couple. She also involved the GP in a referral to a local psycho-geriatric assessment unit which diagnosed Stanley as having multi-infarct dementia. Assistance by way of regular support from a community psychiatric nurse was initially provided to Stanley and Grace, and Stanley began to attend a local day centre, to provide him with some interests outside the home and some respite for Grace. An offer of future contact with the social worker should the need arise was maintained.

Over a period of time Stanley's condition worsened until he reached a point of believing that he was living in the trenches of the war once again. Disagreements with Grace resurfaced and indeed became much more frequent and severe, largely focused on Stanley's personal hygiene, or lack of it. As Stanley firmly believed that he was in the trenches, he was also convinced that there were no bath or toilet facilities for him to use, nor was he willing to change his clothes. One day Grace lost her temper with Stanley' over his refusal to wash, and they both became physically violent.

What is known about elder abuse?

Elder abuse and neglect is a complex and sensitive area to investigate satisfactorily (as are both child abuse and domestic violence). Comparative and developmental norms are much more difficult to establish for older people than with children who have been abused, for example (Bennett, 1990). This means that there are a number of difficulties in attempts to establish the exact nature of the problem. In an early publication, Cloke (1983) characterised these problem areas as:

- definition
- research
- establishing the incidence of abuse and neglect
- determining the causes of abuse
- clarifying the links with other forms of family violence

● acceptance by professionals of the need for procedures to deal with the problem.

Activity 11.1

Think back to your work with older people. Have you, in your opinion, come across incidences of elder abuse, and how do you define this phenomenon?

Comment

There is a lack of clarity about the definition of elder abuse, as we shall see. It is also a relatively new area of concern and research in the UK. Reading through the following will help you to put into perspective some of the issues involved.

As the previous points suggest, there have been difficulties in attempting to establish a comprehensive and sound base to the phenomenon of elder abuse. This is in part because of the lack of agreement concerning a standard definition, but also due to very real difficulties in researching the topic (see also Bennett and Kingston, 1993; Ogg, 1993). For instance, many of the research studies which have been carried out consist of samples which have been very small in scale and have tended to concentrate on cases already known to professionals.

Although the phenomenon was identified by English doctors in the mid-1970s (Baker, 1975; Burston, 1977), it was not until the mid-1980s that the issue was really picked up on in the UK. By contrast, in the USA the issue was identified from the mid-1970s, and began to be researched from that time in an attempt to elucidate the problem and to provide solutions to it.

Causation of elder abuse

It appears unlikely that any one factor causes abuse, but rather that there is an interplay between a number of different factors. There are many possible reasons why abuse happens. Box 11.1 illustrates a number of factors which may be implicated in the development of abuse.

A number of additional risk factors have also been identified, including such aspects as the inability of a carer to care for the older person, other stressors within the family system (for example, unemployment, finance, overcrowding) and inadequate support systems.

Box 11.1   Factors leading to abuse

- a history of long-standing poor relationships within the family (Fulmer and O'Malley, 1987; Homer and Gilleard, 1990)
- the dependency of the abuser on the victim for finance (Hwalek et al., 1986), accommodation and transport (Pillemer, 1986) or emotional support
- the abuser having a history of mental health problems or a substance misuse problem (Pillemer and Wolf, 1986)
- a pre-existing pattern of family violence (inter-generational transmission of violence) (Pillemer and Suitor, 1988)
- the social isolation of the victim and the abuser (Pillemer and Wolf, 1986).

The conceptual frameworks regarding the possible causes of family violence which have been developed so far include a number of distinct theories drawn from the disciplines of psychology, sociology and feminism. Common themes which appear in all forms of family violence, albeit to differing degrees, include: power, gender relations, stress, isolation, and diminished resources (emotional or physical) with which to counter such difficulties.

It is worth noting, however, that such areas have not yet been fully tested to establish their applicability in this country or within elder abuse and neglect. Clearly, a lot more work needs to take place within this area before it is possible to be more certain about the causation of different forms of family violence.

Management of abusive situations

Interventions within abusive situations have recently begun to be developed within the UK. Many strategies have focused on the provision of practical support and assistance (DoH and SSI, 1993). The provision of respite care services, alternative accommodation (either temporary or permanent), counselling for individuals or the family as a whole, or even legal remedies to resolve situations may well prove to be essential strategies. Separation of individuals has been considered as a last resort (DoH and SSI, 1992), and where it does occur may often entail the elderly person entering some form of institutional care (Bennett et al., 1997). A range of interventions with those who abuse, such as treatment for substance abuse or techniques to enhance anger management, are likely to be necessary (Penhale, 1993; Reay, 1997).

The development of assessment protocols to assess the extent of risk within situations is also a necessary component of responding to elder abuse and neglect. Guidance from the Social Services Inspectorate for England and Wales concerning the implementation of the community care reforms implored practitioners to adopt an approach of assessing the needs of individuals (and in particular the social care needs) rather than assessing needs for service provision and for specific services (SSI, 1991). The SSI document, *No Longer Afraid*, concerning elder abuse and neglect, provides a clear statement that the protection of vulnerable elders should not be viewed or treated in isolation from the processes of assessment and care management (SSI, 1993).

The first stage is the assessment process, which should be holistic and needs-led, but abuse-focused if necessary (Bennett et al., 1997). There is likely to be a need for a full consideration of the abusive situation and how to effect lasting change, if possible, within that setting. Safety planning for those individuals who require protection is an essential next step. An appropriate level of risk management also needs to be established once the risk assessment has identified the degree of risk.

Assessment processes are likely to vary between practitioners, and in ideal circumstances should encompass a multidisciplinary approach (DoH and SSI, 1993). Ideally, as with child protection, skilled and qualified practitioners should undertake the most complex and difficult work. Appropriate areas for assessment are contained in Box 11.2.

A number of assessment protocols are now becoming available for use in the UK, although these have largely been developed in the USA (Quinn and Tomita, 1986; Breckman and Adelman, 1988). In addition, there is increasing information on how to ask difficult questions in a sensitive and appropriate manner (for example, Breckman and Adelman, 1988). What also needs to be adequately addressed within such frameworks is a full assessment and appropriate management of risk factors and risky situations.

A focus on the needs of the individual for protection within the assessment process and subsequent care planning stage should not prevent the empowerment of the individual. This would rather ensure that the focus is properly centred on the individuals, the abusive situation (or allegation) and the factors and circumstances which contribute to the situation. The full assessment of needs, including needs for safety, protection and assistance and how best to meet them, forms an essential part of the process. Training courses for professionals are increasingly beginning to focus on such areas in order to assist with appropriate training in assessment and intervention skills. Further development is also necessary in connection with the assessment of risk and dangerousness as a crucial part of the assessment process.

Box 11.2   Areas for assessment

- the abuse (or abusive situation), including antecedents, consequences and likely future patterns
- the individual's methods of dealing with the situation (including any ineffective coping strategies)
- degrees of disability, nature of any dependency (of abuser and abused person)
- risk factors, including stressors, both internal and external to the situation
- family history, social context of the family and dynamics of family relationships within the situation, including information on the balance of power and of communication systems and interactions
- the views, beliefs and attitudes of key players within the situation regarding the nature of the situation and likely outcomes
- consideration of the needs of all parties within the situation is likely to be necessary; it may not be appropriate or necessary to offer an abuser a separate assessment in every situation, but this aspect will require careful consideration; in any case, an assessment of the distinctive needs of all parties will require integration into the overall assessment process.

It is clearly necessary for practitioners to be trained in assessing the risks contained within situations, including risks associated with dangerousness. In addition, practitioners need knowledge concerning which interventions may be required to manage and contain those risks and to provide solutions which are as effective as possible. Practitioners and their managers require skill and expertise in risk management beyond a knowledge and understanding of the factors involved.

Elderly people and their carers generally have the right to refuse intervention in most situations; it is rarely possible to force people to accept intervention. Use of the legal system within situations of abuse may appear to be an extreme option, particularly if the evidence about the abuse is inconclusive. Practitioners may not wish to risk making a situation worse for an elderly person and their family, and of course there may be a real risk of doing that. An example of this would be where the separation of individuals would deprive the elderly person of an important element of their support network which was not adequately replaced by the provision of a substitute form of care. However, there may be an additional danger that the practitioner colludes with the abuser and allows the abuse to continue through over-identification with the abuser as victim, or fear (of violence from the abuser) or a failure to fully appreciate the nature of the situation and the risks involved for the individuals concerned.

Intervention strategies may be directed at the whole family or individual members of the system (abuser or abused), either separately or together. Any action taken will depend on the views and wishes and needs of the individuals, and should include, where necessary, consideration of the needs of those who are cognitively impaired, the degree of impairment and their decision-making capacity. There should also be full consideration of the risks and levels of dangerousness involved, and what might constitute adequate management of the risk(s) to the individual and others involved in the situation.

Policies and procedures are clearly only the first step in the formulation of responses to the problem. It is not usual for procedures to contain the finer detail of what strategies of intervention should be employed in any given situation. The aim is rather to clarify the expectations and responsibilities of staff in terms of responses in the initial stages of receiving a referral, assessing a situation ('investigation') and the subsequent process resulting from the outcome of the assessment and formulation of the care plan.

Details of procedures concerning strategy meetings, case conferences, 'at-risk' registers and reviews are also likely to be set out, together with statements concerning equal opportunities and support for staff. Guidance documents may be developed to accompany the procedures. These aim to clarify certain areas for staff – for example, concerning identification of the different types of abuse and degrees of severity of situations and to provide additional information and assistance for those using the procedure.

It is important to try to identify the primary or main cause of the abuse in order to target interventions appropriately. For instance, if the abuse is principally due to the stress of caregiving, then the provision of services within the community may be appropriate in order to support, alleviate and monitor the situation. However, if the abuse results from some psychopathology of the abuser, then an approach which provides for treatment of the abuser (for example, treatment for substance misuse) together with any necessary protection of the older person is more likely to be indicated.

The willingness of the parties to engage in interventions is of importance here. Clearly, successfully negotiating the boundary between private and public worlds for individuals can be of significance in determining the outcome of interventions. If an individual is willing to undertake treatment for a problem, then the outcome is much more likely to be successful. The key points in dealing with elder abuse are summarised in Box 11.3.

Box 11.3   Key points about elder abuse

- Elder abuse should be the concern of all who work with older people and their carers
- Practitioners should know about risk factors for abuse
- In situations of long-term difficult relationships, there should be a raised awareness of the possibility of abuse occurring
- In situations of long-term care for people with dementing illnesses which include aggressive behaviour towards caregivers, there should be a raised awareness of the possibility of abuse occurring (this may be mutual or two-way abuse)
- Practitioners should know what their local policies and procedures concerning elder abuse (or abuse of vulnerable adults) are and act on them as appropriate.

CASE STUDY 11.2: STANLEY AND GRACE

The social worker visited Grace and Stanley after the incident and reassessed the situation. Although it was treated within a framework of elder abuse according to the social services department procedures, the situation was recognised as being fraught and complex. A punitive approach was not adopted – the family wanted help, not reprisals or removal. The social worker managed to obtain home care assistance (with specially trained home care assistants) to help Grace in keeping Stanley more or less clean. The community psychiatric nurse altered her focus to trying to help the family reach some understanding about Stanley's illness and helping to manage his behaviour.

Stanley remained living at home for several more months. He was admitted to a psychiatric ward for older people based in the district general hospital as a result of a physical (heart-related) problem following a difficult family Christmas. Stanley had been disturbed, extremely disoriented and very aggressive (verbally and physically) for a continuous period of some ten days. Following their assessment, the multidisciplinary case conference held in the hospital with Grace and her family present recommended that Stanley should be admitted to a specialist nursing home. The social worker helped the family to find a place and obtain help with funding. Stanley moved to the home, and initially appeared to be settling in well; his family were able to visit often and were happy. Within three months of his admission, Stanley had a massive stroke and died in his sleep.

Activity 11.2

Return to Activity 11.1 at the start of this chapter and review your responses.

Comment

It will be interesting to note how different your original responses are from your thinking after reading this chapter. These are matters for reflection and personal development.

Having briefly outlined a number of the more general aspects of elder abuse, it seems appropriate in the next section to move to a consideration of elder abuse in relation to issues surrounding the mental health of those who are abused and of those who abuse. This will concern two main areas: dementia and elder abuse, and abuse and the mental health of caregivers.

Dementia and elder abuse

The first area to consider here is the situation of older people with cognitive impairments, in particular those with dementia. Early research suggested that the dependence of the victim was a risk factor associated with abuse, so it is necessary to consider whether people with dementia and associated mental health problems are more likely to be victims of elder abuse than unimpaired individuals. It is perhaps not surprising, given the previous comments made about lack of research generally in elder abuse, to find that there has been rather limited research in this area (Manthorpe, 1995), and as yet no definite answers concerning this question.

In recent literature a number of examples of elder abuse have been given which include dementia as a component factor (Homer and Gilleard, 1990; Grafstrom et al., 1992; SSI, 1992). Relatively few studies have specifically examined the prevalence of abuse of individuals with dementia by their caregivers, but there have been a small number of studies where some consideration has been given to this area; in general terms, these studies have revealed reasonably high rates of abuse.

Two recent articles in the UK have suggested that rates of abuse among older people with mental health problems, in particular those relating to dementia, are higher than would generally be expected from the overall population of people over 65 years old (Wilson, 1994; Cooney and Howard, 1995).

The first of these was a study which looked at levels of elder abuse among older people using a psycho-geriatric service and living in the community. This was a survey of the perceptions of the staff of the service (from differing professional viewpoints), and did not solely or specifically consider dementia, but rather various mental health conditions occurring in later life. The cases were those already known to the staff involved and reported by them in the study, and limited information was given concerning diagnoses of either cognitive impairments or other mental health conditions. Thus the findings are of limited relevance in this context, although they suggest that the rate of elder abuse is higher for clients of this type of service than for the rest of the older population (Wilson, 1994).

The second article consists of a review of existing knowledge (at that point) concerning elder abuse and dementia (Cooney and Howard, 1995). Some of the studies reviewed by these researchers will be outlined in the following sections. The first such study to be considered is that by Coyne et al. from the USA, who sent out questionnaires to carers who had contacted a free helpline for dementia (Coyne et al., 1993). Of the third of carers who responded (342), some 33.1 per cent (92 carers) stated that they had been physically abused by their relative with dementia. The survey also found that 11.9 per cent of respondents (33 carers) indicated that they had physically abused the person they cared for in a number of different acts (biting, kicking and hitting, for example).

The researchers proposed a strong association between the high physical and psychological demands often experienced by caregivers of individuals with dementia and the occurrence of physical abuse. Those carers who reported involvement in abusive behaviour had been caring for longer periods of time overall, and in addition were caring for longer periods during the day than those carers who did not report abuse.

Within this study there also appeared to be a relationship between those caregivers who had been abusive towards their relatives and those who had themselves been the subject of abuse by their relatives. Slightly over a quarter of those carers who reported being abused (26 per cent) stated that they had been abusive to their relative. By contrast, only 4.8 per cent (10 carers) who had not been abused reported that they had been abusive towards their relative (Coyne et al., 1993). It is possible that aggressive or violent behaviour by the 'patient' might provoke a similar response by the carer, that in effect the abuse is mutual and dual-directional in certain situations.

Certainly, this finding relates to earlier research by Levin et al. colleagues in the UK. This research did not specifically look at elder abuse, but rather considered the situation of families caring for 'confused older people' (Levin et al., 1989). One of the key findings, however, was the high risk to carers of both verbal and physical abuse by the recipient of care. A later Australian study by Cahill and Shapiro asked a group of female carers of people with dementia about physical and verbal abuse and sexual violence by the care recipient (Cahill and Shapiro, 1993). This study consisted of a small sample of caregivers which did not fully consider abuse towards the individual with dementia by the caregiver. Of the 39 respondents, 44 per cent said that pushing and shoving had occurred, whilst 25 per cent stated that hitting and pinching had taken place. With regard to verbal abuse, 61 per cent stated that shouting had occurred, whilst 48 per cent reported verbal threats and swearing.

Likewise, a later American study by Pillemer and Suitor, concerning caregivers of people with Alzheimer's disease, indicated that those carers who were caring for relatives who were violent on occasion were themselves fearful of becoming violent and had violent feelings at times. Although this fear of becoming violent was not significantly different between groups of married and non-married caregivers, spouses were much more likely to report both being violent themselves in response to violence by the care recipient and acting on violent feelings than other caregivers (Pillemer and Suitor, 1992).

Within this study, violence also appeared to be related to disruptive behaviour by the care recipient and to whether the caregiver and the care-receiver lived together (co-residence). Caregiver distress generally concerning giving care to people with dementia appears to be greatest when the two parties live together, perhaps because stressors, tensions and conflicts are more difficult to avoid due to proximity (George and Gwyther, 1986; Long, 1981). In addition, in Pillemer and Suitor's study both higher levels of stress and greater degrees of opportunity from more frequent, perhaps unavoidable, contact seemed to contribute to the relationship between co-residence and caregiver fear of becoming violent (Pillemer and Suitor, 1992).

There have been a number of other studies concerning the possible links between dementia and elder abuse, and it is worth mentioning several of these. A recent study in the Netherlands found high levels of verbal aggression (30.2 per cent of caregivers stated they had been verbally aggressive), whilst 10.7 per cent of responding caregivers reported that they had been physically aggressive towards the person with dementia whom they cared for (Pot et al., 1996). Both types of aggression appeared to be related to living in the same household as the person they were caring for and caring for a male. Further, that both types were positively related to caring for an elderly person with higher levels of cognitive impairment and physical dependence (Pot et al., 1996). In addition, verbal aggression was associated with providing higher levels of care, whereas physical aggression appeared to be more related to caring for a spouse and to a higher number of 'psychological complaints' in the caregiver (the study forming part of a longitudinal study of the psychological complaints of informal carers of people with dementia).

This study aimed to compare the situations of those caregivers who reported verbal aggression with those who reported physical aggression. The comparative element of the study considered differences between caregivers in relation to a number of factors: demographics (of caregivers and those with dementia), the psychological complaints of the caregiver and the characteristics of the care recipient. The study determined that physical aggression did differ from verbal aggression in a number of ways, and should not therefore be considered as just an extension of verbal aggression. Differing strategies of intervention appeared to be necessary – for example, attempting to reduce the psychological complaints of the caregiver and the amount of 'burnout' within situations of physical aggression. Further studies replicating such findings from differing cultural perspectives comparing different groups of caregivers who act abusively would clearly be of value. In particular, consideration of what might assist in resolving such situations would be beneficial.

Australian research by Kurrle et al. also determined that within their sample, 46 per cent of those abused had significant dementing illness, whilst some 65 per cent had major disabilities (Kurrle et al., 1992). A further Australian study of importance is that reported by Sadler and colleagues which took place in the same region of Australia as that of Kurrle (Sadler et al., 1995). This study attempted a case-control methodology (considered more reliable in research terms), and reported on 54 cases of abuse and 100 people with dementia who had not been abused. All of the individuals studied were clients of a particular rehabilitation and aged care service. The study appeared to confirm the existence of a strong link between dementia and elder abuse.

When dementia was present with other predisposing factors such as substance abuse or psychiatric illness on the part of the carer, or pre-existing family conflict, then there was a significant risk of abuse happening. The mere presence of dementia, even with the existence of disturbed and aggressive behaviour on the part of the person with dementia, did not appear to result in a higher risk of either psychological or physical abuse for the person with dementia. However, carers did appear to be at risk of physical and/or psychological abuse (Sadler et al., 1995).

In the UK, Homer and Gilleard in their wider 1990 study of a population which had regular respite care from a geriatric service reported that 45 per cent of carers indicated that they had abused their relative. Of this 45 per cent, some 14 per cent admitted to physical abuse. Of the older people receiving the respite service, around 40 per cent had been diagnosed as having dementia. This study found no particular association between a diagnosis of dementia or the degree of impairment and abuse; this is perhaps consistent with other research findings within the field of elder abuse which indicate that the characteristics of abusers are of more relevance than those of the 'victim' (Pillemer and Wolf, 1986).

The study did find that violence (or threat of violence) by the person with dementia seemed to lead to a violent response by the caregiver (Homer and Gilleard, 1990). This led to the suggestion by the researchers that it was disturbed and disruptive behaviour by the care recipient which was likely to result in abuse by the caregiver, rather than simply the presence of cognitive impairment such as dementia.

The finding that those carers who reported being physically abusive to the person they cared for were more likely to report abuse of themselves by that person has also been duplicated in those studies already mentioned, by Coyne et al. (1993) in America and Sadler et al. (1995) in Australia. This suggests a degree of consistency, despite cultural variability and the fact that differing populations were studied. One interpretation is that the presence of abusive or aggressive behaviour by the person who is cognitively impaired is a risk factor for the development and perpetuation of abusive situations. Further research would assist in determining whether this finding holds across other cultures (for example, in less developed countries, or in the Far East) and whether there are any other variables of significance which need to be taken into account.

A further UK study focused on asking carers of people with dementia about the possible occurrence of physical and verbal abuse and neglect of the person they were caring for. This was achieved by way of anonymous questionnaires which were distributed by a voluntary organisation for carers of individuals with dementia and completed by carers (Cooney and Mortimer, 1995).

Although there was a relatively low overall response rate (33.5 per cent), of those who replied, 55 per cent admitted to being involved in at least one type of abuse, with verbal abuse being the most common. Verbal abuse appeared to be linked with the degree of social isolation of the carer and with an existing poor relationship; it also appeared to be a risk factor for physical abuse. Those carers who scored highly on the General Health Questionnaire (measuring psychological health of carers: in this case carers in poorer psychological health) and who had been caring for longer periods appeared to be most at risk of abusing the person they were caring for. Within this study, other variables such as satisfaction with the services provided and amounts of both informal and formal support did not appear to be related to abuse (Cooney and Mortimer, 1995).

There seemed to be some evidence supporting reciprocity of abuse, in that carers who admitted to either physical or verbal abuse were also more likely to report concurrent abusive behaviour of a similar type by the care recipient. Caution should be exercised in relation to his latter finding, as the response rate was low and the sample was therefore small. In addition, the reports by carers were not substantiated at all in any objective sense. Such 'patient' variables as degrees of physical dependency or behaviour and mood disorder did not appear to be significant as no difference was found between individuals who had been abused and those who had not. This suggests some discrepancy between the perceptions of the carers and the actual behaviour of the individual; the researchers were aware of this limitation of the findings (Cooney and Mortimer, 1995).

Abuse and mental health

Much of the research attention in this area appears to have focused on the possible relationships between the psychological and emotional ill health of caregivers and elder abuse. Some of the most well-known research in this field is that conducted in the USA which discovered that 38 per cent of the abusers in the sample had a history of mental ill health, and that 46 per cent of abusers reported a recent decline in their mental health (Wolf and Pillemer, 1989). Psychological and physical abuse appeared to be most closely related to the deterioration in health of the caregiver (mental and physical).

This finding appears consistent on an international basis: from the UK, one small sample of 11 cases of abuse found that 3 of the abusive caregivers had a problem of mental ill health (Clarke and Ogg, 1994), whilst Cooney and Mortimer found that caregivers who admitted being physically abusive in their sample had significantly higher rates of poor psychological health than non-abusive caregivers (Cooney and Mortimer, 1995). Research in Sweden indicated that some 15 per cent of abusers had mental health problems (Saveman and Norberg, 1993). As indicated earlier, recent research in the Netherlands also indicates that physical aggression by caregivers towards care recipients who had dementia appeared to be associated with a higher degree of psychological disturbance on the part of the caregiver, as well as caring for a spouse (Pot et al., 1996).

Canadian research also supports the evidence concerning the mental distress of abusive caregivers. Research by Podnieks indicated that within her sample, 56 per cent of spouses who were physically abusive had psychiatric or emotional problems, compared with 3 per cent of spouses who were not abusive. Those spouses who were abusive were also much more likely to report serious problems with their physical health: 70 per cent, compared to 33 per cent of non-abusers (Podnieks, 1990).

The original study by Homer and Gilleard also reported a finding of note in this regard. Those caregivers who admitted to physical and verbal abuse were significantly more likely to be depressed than those caregivers who were not involved in abusive situations (Homer and Gilleard, 1990). This finding has been repeated in several other studies (Paveza et al., 1992; Coyne et al., 1993).

In addition to this, a great deal of information collated over the past two decades is available concerning the stressful effects of caregiving, especially in relation to caring for people with dementia. A useful review of the psychiatric and physical effects of caregiving in situations of dementia, albeit not specifically concerning elder abuse, has recently been provided (Schulz et al., 1995). What is not wholly clear, however, is the exact nature of the relationship between caregiving and stress, let alone stress, caregiving and abuse.

When considering the stress of caregiving and the possible relationship between this and the aetiology of abusive situations, it is necessary to consider several pertinent factors. First, despite an early and possibly enduring perception that much elder abuse was caused by the stress of caring, it is apparent that there are many dependent older people who are cared for who are not abused even when the caregiving experience is stressful. An explanation which focuses on the differences between abusive and non-abusive situations clearly needs to be developed.

Coupled with this, there needs to be a disaggregation of the apparent linkage between caring, stress and abuse. There seems to have been a tendency for practitioners to over-readily identify with those people who abuse and to consider such individuals as victims in their own right (see also Phillipson and Biggs, 1995, in connection with this). Whilst this might be an appropriate response to some of the situations encountered, as a blanket response by the caring professions ('the poor carer') it is less than helpful. If the aetiology of abuse is reconsidered to examine the nature of power within the dynamic of abusive relationships adequately, such an over-facile and simplistic approach is much less likely to occur or hold sway. Abusive situations and the actors within them might then be dealt with more effectively, although none the less sensitively.

Second, there has been a tendency to equate stress with high levels of physical dependency, which has failed to adequately examine the potential importance of such factors as psychological and emotional dependency within abusive situations (Nolan, 1993). This also links to two further facts: that not all caregivers within such situations of high physical dependence report high stress levels (Nolan, 1993), and that not all people who are very dependent physically are abused or neglected, as would be expected if a straightforward causal relationship were in operation.

Third, research conducted by Steinmetz indicates that it is the perception of the situation by the caregiver as stressful which appears to correlate with the existence of abusive situations, rather than stress *per se* (Steinmetz,

1990). If situations which do not appear, in an objective sense, to be likely to produce high levels of stress are perceived as stressful by the caregiver, then high levels of stress are likely to be experienced and abusive situations may well develop or continue to exist. Whilst stress may indeed contribute to the development and continuation of abusive situations, it appears insufficient, in isolation, to provide a satisfactory explanation for the majority of situations of elder abuse and neglect.

A great deal of the early research within the field of elder abuse set out to determine the 'typical characteristics' of victims of abuse, resulting in some unfortunate stereotypes (Lau and Kosberg, 1979; O'Malley et al., 1984; Penhale, 1992). Subsequent research has focused on establishing profiles of those who abuse. Whilst similar suggestions may be made concerning stereotypes, such research has, in our view, been of value in that it has produced useful information with regard to the psychopathology of a reasonable proportion of those individuals who act abusively. Further, it has indicated that there are likely to be a number of individuals who take on caring roles who are wholly unsuited to such tasks: practically, psychologically, emotionally and physically unsuited to caring. No doubt people take on such roles for a variety of reasons, and some are willing to do so, whilst some are not.

For those people with existing or previous mental health or emotional problems, personality or relationship difficulties, the tasks associated with caring may prove too exacting. A deterioration in their own health or that of the person they care for, or indeed additional complicating factors acting as general contributors in the situation, may lead to the development (or continuation) of an abusive relationship. Reductions in the overall availability and amount of welfare provision to assist such situations will obviously not help in the alleviation and resolution of such problems.

As seen earlier, it is possible that difficult, provocative, even aggressive behaviour by the care recipient may be a contributory factor within the development or continuation of abusive reactions by the caregiver. Similar mechanisms may well be present whether the care recipient has a severe mental illness, a severe learning disability or is significantly cognitively impaired due to a dementing illness. In addition, given the possibility of aggressive or violent behaviour by disturbed individuals, it is clearly quite possible that a mutually abusive relationship may exist or develop within such situations. The findings of Sadler et al. reported earlier suggest that it may be more likely that the existence of other predisposing factors, such as a history of family conflict, or psychopathology on the part of the abuser, is of more importance in the development of abuse (Sadler et al., 1995). Such discrepancies in the findings of different studies in part amplify some of the complexities of the field in general. They are also indicative that no one factor in itself provides adequate explanation, but that a number of factors appear to interrelate and to exist at the same time in many situations.

Concluding comments

There is no absolute evidence that dementia results in elder abuse, although clearly it is an important factor in the development and perpetuation of a number of abusive situations. Research has been rather limited in this area (as with much elder abuse and neglect), and some studies rely on reports by carers or professionals of limited types of abuse or somewhat non-specific mental health difficulties, or are not methodologically sound. These can hardly be considered to be conclusive, but they do present findings which need to be followed up by further research in order to fully test their validity.

Whilst the exact nature of the link between dementia and abuse and the degree of importance of dementia are as yet uncertain, it nevertheless appears that those individuals with dementia who become aggressive and/or violent may well be at increased risk of being abused themselves. This may often occur within the context of a mutually abusive relationship. The risk of abuse for those people with dementia appears to be particularly high in the presence of other predisposing factors such as a history of problematic relationship(s), of substance misuse or psychiatric illness on the part of the carer. Increased vulnerability also seems to be of importance within this multi-factor context. The research evidence that those individuals who abuse are more likely to have mental health (including personality disorders) or substance misuse problems is somewhat more convincing at present.

12 Networks and community interventions

Introduction

This chapter follows on from Chapter 10 concerning groupwork and links with Chapter 13, which present empowerment approaches. There are great similarities between groupwork and networks/community groups. They are separated here to help illustrate the importance of the smaller, more focused use of groups to achieve change and, in the context of this chapter, a common quest for wider social action and change. The main link is the carer support group, in which people with a common interest share information, support one another and, at times, seek development and change in the services provided. Smaller-group work and community-focused approaches are based on the principles of empowerment, participation and strengths.

In this chapter we will provide an overview of community work and networks with respect to people with dementia and their carers. This will focus on two separate but interrelated aspects of the work: actions taken by individual members of the community organising on their own behalf to meet common needs, and actions undertaken by professional workers assisting members of the community with identified needs and concerns.

CASE STUDY 12.1: JEAN

Jean Brown lived on a large council estate to the west of the city. She worked as a cleaner in a nearby pub, getting up at six each day and working from seven until nine each morning. She cared for her father and mother, both of whom were diagnosed as having Alzheimer's disease. Her father had also had a small stroke which had left his speech impaired.

Each day, on her way to work, Jean noticed the church hall, boarded up at the windows, the children's playground and the trail of glass around the swings and, every so often, a burned out car. She knew she was not alone in the area in feeling dismayed at the levels of deprivation and the disenchantment expressed by people in the area. She knew that social services were stretched, and she was grateful for the support she received. A home help came each day to help get her mother and father up in the morning while she was at work, and they each, but separately, attended a day centre once a week. This allowed her to carry on working and to get the shopping in and pay the bills. However, Jean believed more could be done. She wanted to look at other options, even if it meant 'doing it all myself'.

Model and approach

Networks and community groups are a neglected area when working with people with dementia. The positive aspects of social activity, meeting and conversing with others is recognised (Hunter, 1997; Goldsmith, 1996). Social workers are also encouraged under the National Health Service and Community Care Act 1990, the care management approach and, at a different level, when faced with resource constraints to seek alternatives to local authority care and support. Social workers aim to seek the best possible service to meet the client's needs and wishes. This having been said, however, social workers have not used community supports and networks to their full potential.

There may be many reasons for this, including:

- political misgivings about using voluntary and community support at the expense of other necessary services
- a desire not to overburden families and their relatives
- a lack of local agreements and links with communities and groups
- a lack of experience in working with communities
- a lack of knowledge about existing resources
- a lack of resources in the community
- difficulties in relinquishing control to user groups and community groups.

Whatever the reason, the social worker needs to begin to use these valuable resources and services to offer a comprehensive range of interventions to those with dementia and their carers. It is incumbent on social workers in the community to increase their awareness of community resources, to encourage participation and to identify needs. Community social work has never suggested that community organisation and action should replace existing or expensive social care services.

The theoretical underpinning of networking and motivating social support stems from systems thinking (Payne, 1991). The basic ideas of systems thinking state that individuals operate as sub-systems in wider group-living systems – for example, families and partnerships – and wider social systems. Individuals interact with each other and with organisational and wider social systems. Each system, at each level, relies on feedback from or communication with other systems for maintenance and support, and change and growth.

One of the difficulties in defining community work and networking approaches is located in the term 'community'. It has been described as 'those people living within a common geographical area or sharing common interests' (Mayo, 1994), to which Sutton (1994) adds 'individuals sharing a common network or common interpersonal relationships'. It is probably best to adopt a view encompassing elements of all the above. It may be that common interests predominate when working with people with dementia and their carers, and relationships develop from this, but it is unlikely that community social workers will be working with great numbers of people from disparate geographical locations. However the community is defined, the work aims to motivate collective action in response to common needs (Twelvetrees, 1991). It seeks to maximise participation and increase equality of opportunity (Sutton, 1994).

The history of social and community action is long and disparate. It has been promoted by political parties of both Right and Left, but has not been effectively and fully implemented. The reasons for this are manifold but seem to stem from political misgivings concerning power and control, and because priorities demand attention to other actions, such as child protection work (Mayo, 1994).

Following on from Armstrong et al. (1974), Sutton (1994) describes three types of community work commonly undertaken (see Box 12.1).

It is important as a social worker to gain a good awareness of the projects, groups and networks supporting people with dementia. The local Council for Voluntary Service is a good place to start. They may provide a comprehensive list of resources and services in the community, give contact addresses and names or be able to advise where information may be found.

It is also important to have a clear understanding of the work of the national charities and groups working in your area. These may include the Alzheimer's Disease Society, Age Concern and MIND

In each area there are often local theatre groups, local history projects and groups and many lunch clubs attached to churches and other community-based centres. Special interest groups and meetings can be found in most areas, and you may be able to offer advice or point someone in the right direction to gain support and enjoyment. This is equally the case when working with carers as it is when working with the person with dementia. Each person is, as we have said throughout this book, unique and has individual needs. There are groups in the community that will provide an outlet for individuals and their needs if one searches for them.

Box 12.1   Types of community work

- *Community organisation* – this refers to volunteers and local individuals developing self-help projects and attempting to meet identified social needs for themselves. This type of work uses education, participation in initiatives, the publicising of services and the establishment of networks across communities and common interest groups. Payne (1991) adds importantly that it relies on a strengths perspective aimed at improving clients' competence and social functioning
- *Community development* – this is issue-related, such as campaigning for carer support services or on behalf of people with Alzheimer's disease. There is a focused attempt to raise awareness, to campaign and to educate people about their rights
- *Community action* – this type of community work is more overtly political and seeks to challenge existing power structures identified as oppressive.

These three types of work may merge in practice. It may also be the case that community social workers engage more in the latter two types of work, and that volunteers and motivated members of communities engage more in community organisation. This is not necessarily the case, however.

In recent years numerous carer support groups have developed. MIND often offers such groups, as do the voluntary services organisations and many of the statutory sector agencies. Some of these groups offer longer-term support and a social outlet for people.

Undertaking a community profile is an important exercise for community-based practitioners whose remit is to assess and account for the needs of a community (Hawton et al., 1994), but this is no easy or short-term task. It requires intensive planning and arranging. It benefits considerably from the active participation and support of the specified community. For instance, there is no point in simply choosing a 'need' of interest without some indication that members of the community have also identified the need and wish to do something about it. In some geographical areas the needs of carers will receive a higher profile than others. You will first need to know the area well enough to understand how demography affects the needs of that community. Your actions will be guided by this knowledge and by subsequent findings.

ˋCommunity social workers need some skills in collecting information to form an idea about the needs of their area or interest group. A range of interpersonal skills, such as communicating, listening, reflecting and exploring is necessary to develop an understanding of needs. The practitioner also needs to be able to conduct short surveys, to examine the information collected and to analyse the results to identify needs and work out potential strategies with communities to meet those needs. Sutton (1994) provides an excellent introduction to these skills.

The practitioner needs to develop a range of skills. These include liaison, negotiation and communication, co-ordination and management, facilitation, exploration and assessment, providing information, monitoring and evaluating.

The local authority social worker is charged with undertaking comprehensive assessments of need and is likely to have the skills necessary for this kind of work. However, practitioners are charged with undertaking assessments of individuals, families and carers, not communities. It may be that common needs arise when reviewing the assessments undertaken, and a useful and constructive team exercise can be found in identifying common needs and gaps in service provision. Each social services team encompasses a wealth of knowledge and experience. This can be used to identify community groups and voluntary agencies designed to meet needs.

Using community groups and networks opens the day-to-day world to people who have become marginalised and isolated. It helps to re-establish contacts, connections and identities. It is also an empowering way of working that returns an element of control over their lives to the person with dementia and their carer. Whilst resource constraints and statutory service priorities have detracted from the effective promotion of community organisation and action, community work and networking can contribute to processes of change and can develop preventive and participatory approaches to social need.

It is important for social work practitioners to be involved in community organisation and development, and such action is often a great catalyst in moving forward communities which share a common interest. The importance of this approach, lies in the use that those people directly involved can make of it however. It is unlikely to be used by people with dementia because of their widely differing needs and capabilities. Having said this, it is important not to preclude people from action in their communities. An example comes to mind in which a man recently diagnosed with multi-infarct dementia took it upon himself, with the support of others in his interest-community, to set up car maintenance classes for youngsters. His aim was threefold: to enjoy his previous occupation as a mechanic, to give the youngsters something to do and to get him out of the house.

However, most individuals engaging in community organisation and forming helping or supportive networks, will be caregivers. It may be that they will ask for or benefit from practitioner involvement, but this is not necessary. The role of the practitioner may simply be to encourage and provide information when requested to enable like-minded people to meet their needs. Payne (1991) sees the community social worker's role as an intermediary who seeks to foster interdependence among those with common interests and needs.

Activity 12.1

Describe some of the ways in which social workers, people with dementia and their carers might become involved in community work and action. Consider some of the limitations of this kind of work.

Comments

As we saw in Chapter 10, people often come together to pursue a common purpose. This may be a need for services or for advice to assist people living with dementia. The social worker may pursue this need on behalf of people with dementia and their carers, but may be restrained somewhat by the agency role, function, policy and procedure.

Social workers may work best by assisting service users to organise for themselves but perhaps not directly undertaking community work. This will depend on where and for whom the social worker works.

Community-based work and networking is best approached systematically. The following five-step approach works through the identification of need, creating networks and evaluating progress. The value of this approach is that it does not need to be followed by a professional but can be undertaken by any motivated individual who recognises a need in their community. Where dementia is an issue, however, it may be that partnership with professional agencies is important. Caring for someone with dementia can be an extremely emotionally and physically demanding task, and the time required to campaign and establish supportive links may be too much. When local authority social workers cannot offer direct support because of their assessment commitments under the National Health Service and Community Care Act 1990, they may be able to provide links with agencies and organisations in the community who are more attuned to needs and more able to offer the support and help desired:

- **Step one – Identify a need:**
  - Talk with interested parties
  - Discuss with colleagues and agencies
  - Survey needs.

- **Step two – Locate existing support and services:**
  - Survey the area
  - Establish a network of like-minded agencies.

- **Step three – Identify goals:**
  - Convene a network meeting
  - Agree roles and tasks
  - Allocate roles and tasks
  - Agree a timescale for action.

- **Step four – Implement:**
  - Publicise information
  - Target interest groups
  - Maintain communication within the network.

- **Step five – Evaluate:**
  - Evaluate and review.

After the final stage you can see not only whether your goals have been achieved but also whether there is further work to be done. By keeping channels of communication open and by sharing information throughout the network, you create a climate of accountability. People can see what you are doing and what is being achieved.

CASE STUDY 12.2: JEAN
Jean had spoken with her colleague at work, who also looked after her husband after a serious injury at work, and with local shopkeepers and friends in the area. At first this took the form of a general 'moan' about the state of the area, young people and a lack of help and services. It sparked off the germ of an idea, however, which she took to the next review of her mother's and father's home care. She found the social worker to be primarily 'defensive', outlining the reasons why things could not be altered, resource constraints and priorities. By arguing her case, however, Jean

gained the phone number of the local voluntary service organisation, a scheme for youngsters and the caretaker of the church hall she passed each day.

The local volunteer organiser was able to assist her in forming an idea of the needs as she saw them, and gained the support of the social worker to push these ideas forward. Her main needs related to relief and support in caring for her parents – a need she had seen in many others in the area. She also identified the lack of facilities for youngsters. With the help of the volunteer organiser and the support of the social worker, she sought information from others in the area. She did this by knocking on doors and directly asking people what they thought the area needed, then introducing her two main ideas. She also called a community meeting and got her daughter, who worked as a secretary in a local building firm, to take minutes. From this she matched expressed needs against existing services – not only with what was said to be available, but with people's experiences. Whilst the local social services were valued, they were not felt to be adequate. Representatives from the department were asked to participate in group meetings, but after coming to one meeting and seeming to want to take charge, they were not, at this stage, asked to return.

A plan of action was drawn up at the meetings. The volunteer organiser assisted by gaining information, providing advice and working on goals set by the members present. They gained the agreement of the caretaker and church to use the church hall initially as a lunch club, with a view to expanding as a day centre. Local skills were used to ensure the building was safe, clean and practical. Feedback from participants in this work indicated that this was enjoyable and felt worthwhile in itself.

When the church hall was ready to be opened, social services were contacted to ensure that all procedures and regulations had been fulfilled. Some members wanted to bypass this because of their prior experiences but it turned out to be quite profitable. The local social services team offered an advice and welfare benefits slot once a week, and put Jean and the group in touch with other groups in the area which could offer assistance.

As a result, groups of interest to young people were found, and a youth worker became involved more directly with the area.

The lunch group became a day centre, drop-in centre and focus of the local community, and attracted several substantial grants to employ its own community worker. Jean remained active, and the group became a well-known and well-liked complement to existing services and care in the area.

Activity 12.2

Using the five-stage model for community work and planning introduced above, suggest ways in which it might relate to the following
case example.

Jean had noticed that a number of referrals had requested information concerning respite services for people with dementia and carers.
The authority she worked for offered few respite services, and private
and voluntary provision was scarce. Jean consulted with the team
manager after receiving a further request for help, but was told that
social services could do nothing.

Comments

Whilst the social services department and social worker could do
nothing to improve the situation directly, Jean was able to work with
those requesting such services to lobby the local council and agencies
in the area to consider the need for such services. She was able to
identify a wider need, locate a lack of provision and put like-minded
people in touch to pursue a common goal of developing service provision for people with dementia and carers.

Discussion

Community work and the establishment of supportive networks is a demanding task. Community social workers and volunteers undertaking this
work need comprehensive local knowledge, and the trust of local or interested people. The work is political in seeking to achieve change, but is not
aligned to party politics. It is clearly located in the social work values of
choice, participation and empowerment. It seeks to create the conditions of
control within those communities with needs, to allow members of those
communities to determine what goals to pursue, and to give them the
means to do this.

Much of this work with people with dementia and their carers is achieved
by active participation between statutory services, voluntary agencies with
a specific aim of improving care services, support services or information
and getting people involved. It is here that difficulties may arise. The priorities of statutory services relate to the assessment of individual need and
carer need. Local authority social workers do not have the time or resources

to assess community or interest group needs. In this respect care management places the focus on individuals, which can detract from other sources of support.

Where it is possible to identify common needs and where constructive relationships have been established between local authorities and voluntary agencies, it is possible to use the purchaser–provider relationship to ensure that people with common needs are put in touch with relevant organisations in the community. This may in turn lead to the promotion of supportive services and the furtherance of community campaigns alongside the establishment of informal, community-based networks of care, support and information.

13 Empowerment and advocacy

Introduction

The matter of values in practice is fundamental. This is especially the case if the new culture of dementia care (Kitwood and Benson, 1995) or new humanism (Hunter, 1997) is to be achieved. Values in social work practice acknowledge the many levels at which they operate – personal, organisational/agency and societal (Thompson, 1993; Parker, 1995). The principles underlying empowerment, a strengths perspective and advocacy in its many forms operate across these levels and assist in the promotion of rights and responsibilities in dementia care.

This chapter will present a brief review of empowerment in social work practice and discuss advocacy in dementia care. Ways of promoting the rights and responsibilities of all parties to good care will be introduced.

CASE STUDY 13.1: CARL AND MARJORIE

Carl Jordan attended a local authority day centre three days per week. Originally, this had been decided and planned to give his wife, Marjorie, a break from caring and time to shop, clean and see to the house without the seemingly constant demands from Carl. Carl had been consulted and was very willing to go to the centre.

He had been increasingly frustrated at home, since he found it more and more difficult to remember how to complete tasks he found simple in the past. He had worked as a tool operator in a local factory and had enjoyed do-it-yourself activities around the house when he had free time. For the last two years he had been forgetting names and places, and had got up for work and set off to the factory despite having retired eight years previously.

Marjorie teased him at first, but became worried by his behaviour when he became upset and afraid to leave her or let her out of his sight. She felt she could not cope with this, and asked social services for some help. She did not think he would agree to going to a day centre, but when the social worker came to discuss options and possibilities, he appeared very keen on attending.

Marjorie was pleased with the day centre provision, but recognised the stress she had been under and the need for services, information and support. She felt this had not been widely available or publicised, and was angry about this. Carl, on the other hand, was disappointed with the provision. He had met some other men with whom he got on well, but he was bored and felt quite humiliated playing what he saw as children's guessing games and making fancy decorations for the benefit of female staff. Increasingly, he did not wish to go or was rude and verbally aggressive to staff.

The model and approach

Social work has espoused for many years the values of respect for the individual, family, group and community, and promoted commitment to dignity, self-worth and self-determination. This is clear from the writings of Biestek (1961), Hollis (1967) and Timms (1983). Recently, there has been a growing emphasis upon the acceptance and celebration of diversity. This has culminated in anti-oppressive practice which in many ways is akin to the valuing of personhood. One strategy often considered integral to the development of anti-oppressive practice is that of empowerment, but we need to be clear what this means.

The idea of 'becoming powerful' means different things to different people at different times and in different locations. The process by which an individual or group becomes more successful at dealing with and comprehending issues that are of importance to them may be construed as a process of empowerment. It can be argued, however, that since it is usually professionals who seek to empower the disempowered, what is actually occurring is no more than another form of oppression (Adams, 1996). Professionals who *have* bequeath something to those who *have not*. Despite the concept being contested, it is of growing importance in social work in the UK.

In recent years the concept of empowerment has come to underpin social policy guidance and legislation. The Children Act 1989 and the National Health Service and Community Care Act 1990 emphasise participation and individual rights. In the development of community care, Chapman (1993) sees a move from the control of resources by professionals to a social care practitioner role that emphasises facilitation, enabling and acting as a resource. The development of client charters for a range of public services also demonstrates a growing trend towards the promotion of user or consumer power. In fact, empowerment has been much associated with the development of welfare consumerism by the New Right. At the same time, it is associated with the user movement in public services. Adams (1996) provides a useful summary of the various ways in which the concept has been used.

Dalrymple and Burke (1995) stress the importance of a clear definition of empowerment because of the differing uses of the term. A useful definition has been provided by Solomon (1976), who sees empowerment as a problem-solving process in which one engages service users. The process aims to counteract the oppressions that have contributed to the development of the experiences and world-views of those who have limited access, or are denied access, to the power structures of society. Empowerment has been defined as:

> the means by which individuals, groups and/or communities become able to take control of their circumstances and achieve their own goals, thereby being able to work towards helping themselves and others to maximise the quality of their lives. (Adams, 1996, p. 5)

Those without power to effect change are therefore to be empowered: they are to be helped to develop the means to effect changes within their own lives. Empowerment theory stresses the mastery of one's environment and acknowledges that social forces can negatively affect an individual's life and life choices. For people with dementia, it is often not only the illness and disability which leads to a lack of control and influence, but the attitude of others, which is instrumental in creating a climate of disempowerment (Goldsmith, 1996). The goal of the empowerment process is for individuals, families, groups and communities to develop an *internal locus of control*, and an *external locus of responsibility*. The individual will be assisted to gain a sense of control over what happens to them in life, and to acknowledge that because of a particular location within and across certain social dimensions, they are not to blame for their powerlessness and oppression. Browne (1995) describes empowerment practice with older women at risk not only of sexism and ageism but of a wide range of oppressions, and suggests empowerment strategies for working with them. In this discussion she examines some of the potential problems with traditional definitions of empowerment.

The views of people with dementia are often overlooked, ignored or assumed not to exist (Goldsmith, 1996). Chapman (1993) acknowledges that empowerment of people with dementia is difficult, but emphasises that this must not become an excuse for believing it to be impossible because the person is dependent or incapable in themselves. In order to work in an empowering way with people with dementia, it is important for social care practitioners to develop an empathic understanding of the world as experienced by the person with dementia. This involves listening and observing, and spending time interpreting and assessing the person's communication. This can be quite demanding on practitioners (Goldsmith, 1996). It certainly requires them to up date their skills in practice, self-reflection and seeking support.

Social work practitioners therefore need to find ways in which power can be increased in people with dementia and their carers. The process concerns the opportunity to make choices and respect for choices when they are made (Goldsmith, 1996; Chapman, 1993). The choices and decisions need not be major; it is the aggregation of choice, decision-making and feelings of being able to influence one's life that enhance the quality of life of the person. Chapman (1993) suggests that an empowerment approach in social work for people with dementia demands a change of thinking which stresses links and networks, powersharing, mutual respect, acknowledgement of agendas and power imbalance and a person-valuing approach. Of course, this accords very well with the value requirements set for social work (CCETSW, 1995) and the values of respect and self-determination running through social work's history (Timms, 1983).

It is important for good dementia care that social workers:

- see the person first, not the dementia
- listen to the person
- observe individuals in their own environments and settings
- spend time assessing and checking understandings with individuals
- spend time reflecting on their own position, views and values
- seek support from others in their team.

In these ways the social worker can plan in partnership with the person to effect changes which he or she wants, that enhance self-esteem and demonstrate respect for continued decision-making. The social worker is also acting as an agency representative. This may at times conflict with the person's expressed wishes. However, by an honest and explicit approach based on the principles of shared problem-solving, the social worker can promote decision-making and self-determination within clearly expressed boundaries. This is the way the adult human world functions, and again, it allows certain levels of control with certain responsibilities.

CASE STUDY 13.2: CARL AND PAUL

Carl's social worker, Paul, visited him at the day centre regularly. He noticed the frustration and the increased verbal outbursts. When speaking to staff at the centre, he was told that Carl was simply a difficult man and they had dealt with 'his sort' before. They told him not to worry because he would soon pass through this phase as he lost more and more of his abilities. Paul was shocked by the attitude of the centre staff, and was determined to seek Carl's views of the situation.

He spent time with Carl at the day centre throughout the day, and learned the routines and general content of activities. Given his knowledge of Carl's background, he began to form a picture of his growing disillusionment. In order to be sure he was 'on the right track', he shared his reflections with Carl. Carl spoke with him about his work and his hobbies and interests. This gave Paul an idea of the kinds of activities which might be more meaningful to Carl. Carl was included in this planning, and wanted to build something and use his interests. Paul checked with staff at the centre whether it would be possible to run a small group for some of the men, building models of past workplaces. This was agreed.

Carl felt useful in sharing some of his previous skills in this group and helping others who were not as accomplished as him. Although he found it difficult to complete things or stay on tasks for long periods, the model-building acted as a focus in which he could direct his understanding, his thoughts and energies and confirm his ability to influence the world around him.

This is a fairly simple example, and one which relies on partnership with professionals. However, it demonstrates how one man was assisted to direct and establish control over an important and self-validating part of his life.

Dalrymple and Burke (1995) emphasise the links between one's personal position and structural inequalities in wider society. For them empowerment is a process and a goal whereby the service user is assisted to take steps to reduce their own powerlessness. Power is, of course, integral to the concept. It can be seen to operate at many levels:

1 *Level of feeling* – having a sense of ownership of one's personal experiences and biography, which can be achieved by affirming and validating the person with dementia.
2 *Level of ideas* – increasing self-efficacy and the ability to produce and regulate events in one's life; this needs greater planning and tenacity, but can be achieved.
3 *Level of action* – ensuring that the formulation and enactment of policy decisions are influenced by those directly affected by them; this is harder to achieve, but can involve all those influenced by the situation, including caregivers.

Activity 13.1

What are some of the important points to remember when working with people with dementia?

Comments

If you are working in an empowering way with people with dementia, you will be actively seeking to return control, to increase power and to ensure that each person's voice is heard. This is important to a culture which values and respects people as unique individuals who interact with one another.

Empowerment strategies for people with dementia are anti-oppressive in that they see the person first, not the disability resulting from the dementia.

Empowerment strategies also ensure that the social worker checks his or her own power and potential for disempowerment. The social worker continually checks his or her understanding, and works at the pace of the service user and on behalf of them. The social worker's mandate comes from the person themselves. Where dementia is an issue, this means listening to what is said, valuing the person with dementia and championing the rights of those disabled by a disease and by society's reactions to it.

This structural and political approach to empowerment stems to a large extent from radical social work (Adams, 1996). It relies on 'cause advocacy' (Payne, 1991), in which people are empowered to campaign for services, resources, choice and rights at a wider level. This is important in relating to work mentioned in Chapter 12 concerning networks. It also relates to the promotion of self-help strategies (see also Mullender and Ward, 1991). When working with people with dementia, however, advocacy at an individual level – 'case advocacy' (Payne, 1991) – is often more immediately effective. It is often difficult for social work practitioners to act as advocates because of the conflict of interest arising from agency requirements and not being able to work in conflict with one's own employing agency (Chapman, 1993). However, independent advocacy schemes are important as they can prevent services and others involved treating the person with dementia as an object without a voice. Social work skills, knowledge and values are important to this role. Independent advocates can promote the needs of the person and take the time necessary to ensure views, wishes and choices are made explicit and heard. The use of independent advocates, although expensive, can also offer a useful counterbalance between the needs of carers and the needs of the person with dementia (Burton, 1997).

Burton (1997) also states that the need for advocacy in dementia care is clear at times of critical transitions such as a move into residential care, while in residential care, for ethnic minority groups, and to ensure that people receive their entitlements as consumers and under the law. Of course, it is not always possible for people to advocate on their own behalf, and questions of ethics and values arise when others are advocating on behalf of the person with dementia. By acting in 'the best interests' of the person, it is easy to argue the practitioner is merely being paternalistic and possibly acting on behalf of his or her agency, rather than the service user. It may be that relying on knowledge of past beliefs and values can provide important information about what the person would wish for now. This may be best achieved by seeking an independent advocate. However, there are also dangers here. The independent advocate may rely on forming an intense and deep relationship with the service user. The need for values and boundaries is important, as such relationships are open to abuse.

CASE STUDY 13.3: CARL

Carl's memory deteriorated over time, and his ability to undertake tasks declined. The model-making group reached a conclusion, and although staff learned to take individual feelings and needs into account more, Carl began to be seen as a placid, undemanding man who retained few skills and abilities. His needs were once again not being met. This time there was no overt attempt by Carl to communicate distress or frustration. He was simply quiet. However, the social services department were running a pilot advocacy scheme for people with dementia, and people in the day centre were considered for inclusion.

Carl was observed to be someone who was losing out on active stimulation because he was quiet and caused no overt problems which got him noticed. An advocate was appointed who looked at his previous history, read the case files, spoke with his wife and family and carers at the day centre, and suggested that he might like to be more actively involved in matters. The advocate sought to find ways of achieving this, and looked towards more individual work, reminiscence and befriending. This resulted in Carl visiting his old factory, the street in which he was born and the local football club. He became more talkative at times and brought up memories of his past work, family and an FA Cup match he attended.

Activity 13.2

Reflect on ways in which you might be able to act as an advocate on behalf of people with dementia or their carers in your work in dementia care.

Comments

Your response will depend on your workplace. As a statutory social worker you may have responsibilities which mean you cannot act as an independent advocate, but you may provide people with the knowledge to gain independent advocacy. You may also work within your authority to increase awareness of the needs of people with dementia.

If you work for a voluntary agency, you may be involved in advocacy on some level, but again, you may have a number of restraints preventing you from adopting a full advocate position.

It is important to know your own role and the values of your job and your profession. In this way, if you cannot act as an advocate you can ensure that information is provided and offered to give people as full a choice as possible.

It is important to remember that it is not only people with dementia who are disempowered. Often carers are isolated and 'trapped' in a world that demands their complete commitment to and concentration on the daily care needs of the person they live with or care for. It is important to ensure that social care services are offered in such a way that real choice is offered, full information is provided and carers are given the right to change their mind. Whilst resource questions limit the choices we have, the element of control is all-important. Carers need to be in control of the care they provide and to have real alternatives available should they so need or wish. Chapman (1993) describes a training course for carers in which education, support and choice was encouraged by a mutual support group which used professionals as a resource for them. This worked well in increasing the perceptions of self-control of the participants.

In order to counter the challenge that empowerment is often the giving of limited power by the powerful, it is important to note that social work itself does not and cannot empower. It can act as a resource committed to people empowering themselves, however. For empowerment practice to work, there needs to be real participation between service users, carers and practitioners (Adams, 1996). This necessarily depends on offering choice and opportunities to make choices, and a redistribution of resources or changes to the way resources are allocated. The most important step forward is involving people with dementia and their carers in a process of consultation.

Cowger (1994) stresses that it is the use of clients' strengths that helps to promote positive empowerment practice and mitigates, to some extent, the unequal power relations between service users and practitioners. He proposes a set of 12 guidelines for assessment that reflect that position:

1 Pre-eminence is given to the service user's understanding.
2 The service user is believed.
3 The service user's wants are determined.
4 Personal and environmental strengths are explored.
5 Assessment of strengths is multidimensional.
6 Uniqueness of the individual is acknowledged in the assessment.
7 Client-friendly language is used.
8 Assessment is conducted as a joint activity.
9 A mutual agreement is reached.
10 Blame and blaming are avoided.
11 Singular cause-and-effect thinking is avoided.
12 The intention is to assess need, not to diagnose deficits.

CASE STUDY 13.4: MARJORIE

Marjorie was able to advocate on her own behalf when she found the stress too intolerable to manage. She was listened to, and respite care was arranged at the local day centre. This achievement encouraged her to meet with other carers and to begin to advocate strongly on behalf of themselves and others caring for people with dementia.

The first social worker, Paul, who had assisted with Carl's model-making project, worked in partnership with Marjorie to campaign for services to be publicised and information to be made available. This initial assistance helped her to feel she could alter situations and achieve ends herself. This helped her to organise carers, and for them to determine what they felt they needed and to plan how they would put their case to doctors, social workers and voluntary agencies in the area.

Marjorie was asked to contribute to the local authority community care plan for the following year.

In working with people with dementia and carers, it is advantageous to form participatory alliances where possible and to work with their strengths. This 'strengths perspective' is taken up by Saleeby (1996), who believes this is important in giving people control, working in partnership and encouraging interdependence. Concentrating on people's strengths does not deny the reality of difficulties and deficits arising from their disability, but it starts where they are able to, and encourages and promotes choice and opportunity according to the individual's wants, wishes and needs.

It can be argued, however, that whilst the values and principles under-pinning empowerment are accepted, the realities of practice – often with unwilling and involuntary clients – make such a process redundant.

Can we work in empowering ways with involuntary clients? If we are honest in our assessment and about our role, explaining the reasons for our involvement as clearly as possible, it may be that we can reach agreement with service users concerning elements of our intervention. Often end-goals are shared. If the goals are held in common, there is the possibility of negotiating the processes to achieve these. People with dementia may not wish our involvement, may not see any reason for concern. Carers may believe too little is being done to help them or to 'make' the person they care for accept services. Working together in participation with service users and carers may lead to a change in focus from voluntary and involun-tary service users to a mutual striving to achieve change. This commitment to empowerment works at the level of practice with individuals. The value of empowerment can also be seen in wider terms. Working with clients to counteract disadvantage, to acknowledge and work to rectify the negative effects of social structures and dimensions represents a legitimate social work role. Of course, in practice the work with individuals and small living groups forms the bulk of one's endeavours. However, in liaison with the variety of agencies often involved in social care and social regulation, op-portunities exist for promoting more positive approaches to the regulation of social life that encourages the sharing of power and development of user involvement at all levels.

Summary

It is important to promote practice which involves, includes and affirms the worth of people with dementia and their carers. This is clearly the intention of empowerment strategies. In the world of social services and care man-agement, the potential for conflicts of interest must be recognised, but the challenge of empowerment, advocacy and the affirmation of people with dementia must continue. In this chapter we have reviewed empowerment approaches and advocacy, examining how they might be used for people with dementia and their carers.

Epilogue

Social workers practise in a changing environment. This has always been the case throughout the profession's short history, and will no doubt continue to be so. Legislation and policy develops as society adapts to changing experience, values and needs. Departmental and local government reorganisations happen frequently. All these factors have an impact on the way social workers approach their clients and what they do with them. In specific terms, these social and organisational influences have an impact on the way social workers practise with people with dementia and their carers.

It is imperative that social work carves out a clear role in the context of care management and the provision of social services and care for people with dementia. There is increased evidence from practice that approaches which value the personhood of those people worked with encourage and promote quality of life and participation. The new culture of dementia care is developing theoretically and in practice. This is shown clearly in Kitwood's exposition of the subject (Kitwood, 1997b).

It seems likely that adult social services, including social work for people with dementia, will increasingly be provided from a mixed economy of care. Whilst local authority social workers will assess and commission services, they may not always be the ones who provide the services. These may come from a variety of voluntary and private agencies. These agencies are employing people qualified in health and social care work. In this context, a commitment to respect for the person and citizenship is essential. This can be achieved by the judicious employment of the methods and approaches we have outlined throughout this book.

The approaches discussed are tools to be used by people involved with other human beings. They are only as 'good', in ethical terms, as the values which lie behind their use. However, they provide keys to effective practice which can validate the social and individual worth of the person. Indi-

211

vidual characteristics also play a large part in any interpersonal interaction. The models and approaches are affected by the social workers' qualities and personalities, and those of the clients. When all these factors are taken into account and the issues for work are recognised and agreed, the best possible way forward for social work practice can be pursued.

There is a stigma attached to involvement with social workers. This may stem from a variety of sources, including the media presentation of social workers as threatening the private life of families, their association with placing people in long-term residential care and their perceived ineffectiveness. People are therefore only likely to call upon the services of a social worker at a time of crisis (Parker, 1992). Working with people at a point of crisis, when their usual 'tried and tested' methods of coping no longer achieve their goals, often forms the initial point of entry for a social worker into a family's life. Working with crisis allows those involved time to reflect, to consider options and alternatives, and to agree a longer-term plan of action to meet identified needs. It is the starting point for a variety of interventions. Some of these may be practice-based, but some may relate to working with individuals to develop more systematic responses to people that promote their rights and recognise their responsibilities. It is from the perspective of crisis that a clear, interventive strategy can often be formulated.

The second part of the book has outlined three broad areas in which social workers may work to promote citizenship, coping and quality of life. These involve action-oriented approaches that are often directive but are based on the concepts of partnership, agreement and respect for the client. There are also listening approaches that emphasise more the counselling skills so necessary to any interpersonal work. People do not live in a vacuum, and wider social issues often need to be taken into account. The support of friends, like-minded individuals and community groups is important in developing attitudes and approaches which maximise quality of life and respect for persons.

There is often disagreement among practitioners about the best, most effective methods to be used. There are different theoretical perspectives to be taken. Whilst eclecticism has rightly been criticised as contradictory and confusing on a theoretical level, the use of a range of approaches can often enhance practice. An overall approach based on values and a fundamental approach to people based on partnership, shared learning and growth sits well with counselling and listening approaches, and action approaches based on social learning theories. In fact, the skills involved in interpersonal work are the same as those required for cognitive-behavioural and task-centred interventions, and these approaches together often underlie wider community-based approaches.

The plan for work needs to take into account, first of all, needs identified by the person with dementia and his or her carers. It is also dependent upon the working brief of the social worker involved. For instance, a commissioner of services or an assessment officer may take a different approach to a care manager, residential care worker or day care worker. The context of work influences the intervention.

Cognitive-behavioural approaches and task-centred work have been criticised for being too directive, sometimes too powerful and as inappropriate for people who can no longer make connections and solve problems. In fact, these approaches champion such ideals as partnership, the development of new skills, and enhancing existing skills and behaviours within the particular context in which the individual lives. Whilst it is certainly true that new learning can often be more difficult and sometimes not possible, each individual is unique and has their own learning capacity. Also, people are social beings, and many have other people around them who can alter and adapt their own approaches to the person they care for. This can reap tremendous benefits. Action-based approaches demand commitment and motivation from all parties. They are about increasing rather than restricting life chances and opportunities, and are consonant with the values of respect and dignity of the person.

In working with people with dementia and carers, it is important to validate the feelings and emotions people express. Time is needed for people to work through the enormity of situations and to work out the meanings for them of dementia and caregiving. The use of counselling and psychotherapeutic approaches, once thought to be irrelevant for people with dementia, is now recognised as important to well-being and essential to the maintenance and preservation of a sense of self-identity and respect. Individual counselling, reminiscence work and groupwork are part of the large array of positive interventions which can be brought to social work for people with dementia.

Whilst most of the techniques discussed relate to interpersonal work and work in family or caregiving situations, this is not all that social workers do. There is a wider community angle in which social work participation can be effective. Social workers have a key role in dealing with elder abuse. This concerns intervention on an interpersonal and at a service level, but also necessitates involvement in social education and awareness-raising, liaison with other professionals and the development of effective policies and procedures to deal with this phenomenon. The skills of negotiation, liaison, people management and policy development are also important to community work and development and empowerment approaches. Ageism in all its forms – devaluing work with older people, older people with mental health problems and disabilities, economic and political invalidation – has contributed to the present state of affairs in which people's awareness of their own and other people's value and worth needs to be reaffirmed.

The common theme running through these chapters is optimism. It is an optimism built on recent practice and theoretical developments which emphasise the value and worth of the individual and promote 'personhood'. The techniques are those traditionally employed by social workers in a variety of practice settings. When underpinned by this value base, they fit neatly into the 'new culture of dementia care' (Kitwood and Benson, 1995).

CASE STUDY: GEORGE

In 1966 George's mother came to stay with his family. She was recently widowed, 83 years old, and prone to forgetfulness and wandering. The strain on the family was great. Friends stopped visiting because of George's mother's garbled interruptions in their conversations. George's wife became depressed at having to 'spend all day looking after that woman'. After six months they asked for her to be put in a residential home. She died three months later.

In 1995 George suffered a stroke. He had been suffering from Alzheimer's disease for two years, according to his doctor. George's wife, Mary, was physically frail but wanted to care for him as long as she could. The family discussed options with the social worker. George was included, and his views were sought at each stage of the process. A care plan was devised which detailed the care and support George and Mary were to receive. They made an agreement with the social worker about this. After six months, Mary died. George was consulted about his wants and wishes, and the social work support he had been receiving helped him to determine to stay at home, supported by people he had come to *know* and trust.

References

Adams, R. (1996) *Social Work and Empowerment*, Basingstoke: Macmillan.

Aguilera, D.C. (1990) *Crisis Intervention: Theory and Methodology* (6th ed.), St Louis, MI: C.V. Mosby.

Aguilera, D.C. and Messick, J.M. (1974) *Crisis Intervention: Theory and Methodology*, St Louis, MI: C.V. Mosby.

Aguilera, D.C. and Messick, J.M. (1982) *Crisis Intervention Therapy for Psychological Emergencies*, New York: Plume.

Allen, I., Hogg, D. and Peace, S. (1992) *Elderly People: Choice, Participation and Satisfaction*, London: Policy Studies Institute.

Arber, S. and Ginn, J. (1991) *Gender and Later Life*, London: Sage.

Arean, P.A., Perri, M.G., Nezu, A.M. and Schein, R.L. (1993) 'Comparative effectiveness of social problem-solving therapy and reminiscence therapy as treatments for depression in older adults', *Journal of Consulting and Clinical Psychology*, 61, 1,003–10.

Armstrong, R., Davies, C., Doyle, M. and Powell, A. (1974) *Case Studies in Community Work*, Vol. 1, Manchester: Manchester Monographs.

Audit Commission (1986) *Making a Reality of Community Care*, London: HMSO.

Audit Commission (1992) *The Community Revolution*, London: HMSO.

Bachar, E., Kindler, S., Schefler, G. and Lerer, B. (1991) 'Reminiscing as a technique in the group psychotherapy of depression: A comparative study', *British Journal of Clinical Psychology*, 30, 375–7.

Baker, A.A. (1975) 'Granny bashing', *Modern Geriatrics*, 5, 8, 20–4.

Baldwin, B.A. (1979) 'Crisis intervention: An overview of theory and practice', *The Counseling Psychologist*, 8, 43–52.

Baldwin, B.A. (1981) 'Crisis intervention: An overview of theory and practice', in Burgess, A.W. and Baldwin, B.A. (1981) *Crisis Intervention Theory and Practice: A Clinical Handbook*, Englewood Cliffs, NJ: Prentice-Hall.

Bandura, A. (1977) *Social Learning Theory,* Englewood Cliffs, NJ: Prentice-Hall.

Barclay Report (1982) *Social Workers: Their Role and Tasks,* London: Bedford Square Press.

Barth, R.P. (1989) 'Evaluation of a task-centred child abuse prevention program', *Children and Youth Services Review,* 11, 117–31.

BASW (1975) *A Code of Ethics for Social Workers,* Birmingham: British Association of Social Workers.

Beck, A.T. (1967) *Depression: Clinical, Experimental and Theoretical Aspects,* New York: Harper and Row.

Beck, A.T. (1970) 'Cognitive therapy: Nature and relationship to behavior therapy', *Behavior Therapy,* 1, 184–200.

Beck, A.T. (1976) *Cognitive Therapy and the Emotional Disorders,* New York: International Universities Press.

Benbenishty, R. and Ben-Zaken, A. (1988) 'Computer-aided process of monitoring task-centred family interventions', *Social Work Research and Abstracts,* 24, 7–9.

Benbow, S.M. (1997) 'Therapies in old age psychiatry: Reflections on recent changes', in Marshall, M. (ed.) *State of the Art in Dementia Care,* London: Centre for Policy on Ageing.

Bender, M., Norris, A. and Bauckham, P. (1987) *Groupwork with the Elderly: Principles and Practice,* Bicester: Winslow Press.

Bennett, G.C. (1990) 'Action on elder abuse in the '90s: New definition will help', *Geriatric Medicine,* April, 53–4.

Bennett, G.C., and Kingston, P.A (1993) *Elder Abuse: Theories, Concepts and Interventions,* London: Chapman and Hall.

Bennett, G.C., Kingston, P.A. and Penhale, B. (1997) *The Dimensions of Elder Abuse: Perspectives for Practitioners,* Basingstoke: Macmillan.

Biestek, F.P. (1961) *The Casework Relationship,* London: Allen and Unwin.

Bleathman, C. and Morton, I. (1988) 'Validation therapy and the demented elderly', *Journal of Advanced Nursing,* 13, 511–14.

Bloom, B. (1963) 'Definitional aspects of the crisis concept', *Journal of Consulting Psychology,* 27, 498–502.

Bond, J. (1987) 'Psychiatric illness in late life: A study of prevalence in a Scottish population', *International Journal of Geriatric Psychiatry,* 2, 39–58.

Bond, J., Briggs, R. and Coleman, P. (1990) 'The study of ageing', in Bond, J. and Coleman, P. (eds) *Ageing in Society: An Introduction to Social Gerontology,* London: Sage.

Brandon, D. (1989) 'Who sets the boundaries of control?', *Service Brokerage,* 1, iii.

Breckman, R. and Adelman, R. (1988) *Strategies for Helping the Victims of Elder Mistreatment,* London: Sage.

Brody, C.M. (1990) 'Women in a nursing home: Living with hope and meaning', *Psychology of Women Quarterly*, 14, 579–92.

Bromley, D.B. (1988) *Human Ageing*, 3rd edn, London: Penguin.

Bromley, D.B. (1990) *Behavioural Gerontology: Central Issues in the Psychology of Ageing*, Chichester: John Wiley.

Brown, G.W. and Harris, T.O. (1978) *Social Origins of Depression*, London: Tavistock.

Browne, C. (1995) 'Empowerment in social work practice with older women', *Social Work*, 40, 358–64.

Browne, K. (1989) 'Family violence: Elder and spouse abuse', in Howells, K. and Hollin, C.R. (eds) *Clinical Approaches to Violence*, London: John Wiley.

Browne, K. and Herbert, M. (1997) *Preventing Family Violence*, Chichester: John Wiley.

Buchanan, K. and Middleton, D. (1995) 'Voices of experience: Talk, identity and membership in reminiscence groups', *Ageing and Society*, 15, 457–91.

Burgess, A.W. and Baldwin, B.A. (1981) *Crisis Intervention Theory and Practice: A Clinical Handbook*, Englewood Cliffs, NJ: Prentice-Hall.

Burston, G.R. (1977) 'Granny bashing', *British Medical Journal*, 3, 592.

Burton, A. (1997) 'Dementia: A case for advocacy?', in Hunter, S. (ed.) *Dementia: Challenges and New Directions*, London: Jessica Kingsley.

Butler, J., Bow, I. and Gibbons, J. (1978) 'Task-centred casework with marital problems', *British Journal of Social Work*, 8, 393–410.

Butler, R.N. (1963) 'The life review: An interpretation of reminiscence in the aged', *Psychiatry*, 26, 65–76.

Bytheway, B. (1994) *Ageism*, Buckingham: Open University Press.

Cahill, S. and Shapiro, M. (1993) '"I think he might have hit me once": Aggression towards caregivers in dementia', *Australian Journal on Ageing*, 12, 4, 10–15.

Caplan, G. (1961) *An Approach to Community Mental Health*, New York: Grune and Stratton.

Caplan, G. (1964) *Principles of Preventive Psychiatry*, New York: Basic Books.

Carkhuff, R.R. (1987) *The Art of Helping*, 6th edn, Amherst, MA: Human Resource Development Press.

CCETSW (1995) *DipSW Rules and Requirements for the Diploma in Social Work*, CCETSW Paper 30, London: Central Council for Education and Training in Social Work.

Chapman, A. (1993) 'Empowerment', in Chapman, A. and Marshall, M. (eds) *Dementia: New Skills for Social Workers*, London: Jessica Kingsley.

Chapman, A., Jacques, A. and Marshall, M. (1994) *Dementia Care: A Handbook for Residential and Day Care*, London: Age Concern England.

Chapman, A. and Marshall, M. (eds) (1993) *Dementia: New Skills for Social Workers*, London: Jessica Kingsley.

Cheetham, J., Fuller, R., McIvor, G. and Petch, A. (1992) *Evaluating Social Work Effectiveness*, Buckingham: Open University Press.

Christ, G.H., Moynihan, R.T. and Gallo-Silver, L. (1991) 'Human immuno-deficiency virus and crisis intervention: A task-focused approach', in Roberts, A.R. (ed.) *Contemporary Perspectives on Crisis Intervention and Prevention*, Englewood Cliffs, NJ: Prentice-Hall.

Claridge, G. (1986) *Origins of Mental Illness*, Oxford: Blackwell.

Clarke, C.L. (1997) 'In sickness and in health: Remembering the relation-ship in family caregiving for people with dementia', in Marshall, M. (ed.) *State of the Art in Dementia Care*, London: Centre for Policy on Ageing.

Clarke, M. and Ogg, J. (1994) 'Recognition and prevention of elder abuse', *Journal of Community Nursing*, 8, 2, 4–6.

Clarke-Kehoe, A. and Harris, P. (1992) 'It's the way that you say it', *Community Care*, 9 July, 8–9.

Cloke, C. (1983) *Old Age Abuse in the Domestic Setting: A Review*, Portsmouth: Age Concern.

Clough, R. (ed.) (1996) *The Abuse of Care in Residential Institutions*, London: Whiting and Birch.

Cohen, U. and Weisman, G.D. (1991) *Holding on to Home: Designing Environ-ments for People with Dementia*, Maryland: Johns Hopkins University Press.

Coleman, P. (1987) *Ageing and Reminiscence Processes: Social and Clinical Im-plications*, Chichester: Wiley.

Coleman, P. (1994) 'Reminiscence within the study of ageing: The social significance of story', in Bornat, J. (ed.) *Reminiscence Reviewed: Perspec-tives, Evaluations, Achievements*, Buckingham: Open University Press.

Cooney, C. and Howard, R. (1995) 'Abuse of patients with dementia by their carers: Out of sight but not out of mind', *International Journal of Geriatric Psychiatry*, 10, 735–41.

Cooney, C. and Mortimer, A. (1995) 'Elder abuse and dementia', *International Journal of Social Psychiatry*, 41, 4, 276–83.

Coulshed, V. (1991) *Social Work Practice: An Introduction*, 2nd edn, Basingstoke: Macmillan.

Cournoyer, B. (1991) *The Social Work Skills Handbook*, Belmont, CA: Wadsworth.

Cowger, C. (1994) 'Assessing client strengths: Clinical assessment for client empowerment', *Social Work*, 19, 262–8.

Coyne, A., Reichman, W.E. and Berbig, L.J. (1993) 'The relationship between dementia and elder abuse', *American Journal of Psychiatry*, 150, 4, 643–6.

Cumming, E. and Henry, W. (1961) *Growing Old: The Process of Disengage-ment*, New York: Basic Books.

Dalrymple, J. and Burke, B. (1995) *Anti-Oppressive Practice*, Oxford: Oxford University Press.

Dattilio, F.M. and Freeman, A. (1994) *Cognitive-behavioral Strategies in Crisis Intervention*, New York: Guilford Press.

De Klerk Rubin, V. (1994) 'How validation is misunderstood', *Journal of Dementia Care*, 2, 14–16.

DHSS (1969) *Report of the Committee of Inquiry into Allegations of Ill-treatment and Other Irregularities at Ely Hospital, Cardiff*, Cmnd 3785, London: HMSO.

DHSS (1971) *Report of the Farleigh Hospital Committee of Inquiry*, Cmnd 4557, London: HMSO.

DHSS (1972) *Report of the Committee of Inquiry into Whittingham Hospital*, Cmnd 4871, London: HMSO.

DHSS (1976) *Priorities for Health and Social Services in England*, London: HMSO.

DHSS (1981a) *Care in Action: A Handbook of Policies and Priorities for the Health and Personal Social Services in England*, London: HMSO.

DHSS (1981b) *Care in the Community*, London: HMSO.

Dobroff, R. (1984) 'Introduction: A time for reclaiming the past', in Kaminsky, M. (ed.) *The Uses of Reminiscence: New Ways of Working with Older Adults*, New York: Haworth Press.

Doel, M. (1994) 'Task-centred work', in Hanvey, C. and Philpot, T. (eds) *Practising Social Work*, London and New York: Routledge.

Doel, M. and Marsh, P. (1992) *Task-centred Social Work*, Aldershot: Arena.

DoH (1989) *Caring for People: Community Care in the Next Decade and Beyond*, Cmnd 849, London: HMSO.

DoH (1990) *Community Care in the Next Decade and Beyond: Policy Guidance*, London: HMSO.

DoH and SSI (Department of Health/Social Services Inspectorate) (1993) *No Longer Afraid: The Safeguard of Older People in the Domestic Setting*, London: HMSO.

Dryden, W. (ed.) (1996) *Research in Counselling and Psychotherapy*, London: Sage.

Echlin, R. and Ramon, S. (1992) 'Safe as houses', *Nursing Times*, 88, 38–40.

Edlis, N. (1993) 'Rape crisis: Development of a center in an Israeli hospital', *Social Work in Health Care*, 18, 169–78.

Egan, G. (1990) *The Skilled Helper: A Systematic Approach to Effective Helping*, 4th edn, Pacific Grove, CA: Brooks/Cole Publishing.

Erikson, E. (1950) *Childhood and Society*, London: W.W. Norton.

Fatout, M.F. (1992) *Models for Change in Social Group Work*, New York: Adline De Gruyter.

Feil, N. (1992) *Validation: The Feil Method*, Cleveland, OH: Edward Feil Productions.

Feil, N. (1993) *The Validation Breakthrough*, Baltimore: Health Professions Press.

Finch, J. (1989) *Family Obligations and Social Change*, Cambridge: Polity Press.

Frank, B.A. (1995) 'People with dementia can communicate – if we are able to hear', in Kitwood, T. and Benson, S. (eds) *The New Culture of Dementia Care*, London: Hawker.

Friedman, M. and Friedman, R. (1980) *Free to Choose*, London: Macmillan.

Froggatt, A. (1988) 'Self-awareness in early dementia', in Gearing, B., Johnson, M. and Heller, T. (eds) *Mental Health Problems in Old Age*, Chichester: John Wiley.

Froggatt, A. (1990) *Family Work with Elderly People*, Basingstoke: Macmillan.

Fulmer, T. and O'Malley, T. (1987) *Inadequate Care of the Elderly: A Health Care Perspective on Abuse and Neglect*, New York: Springer Publications.

Galassi, F.S. (1991) 'A life review workshop for gay and lesbian elders', *Journal of Gerontological Social Work*, 16, 75–86.

Gambrill, E. (1994) 'What's in a name? Task-centred, empirical and behavioral practice' *Social Services Review*, 68, 578–99.

Garvin, C. (1992) 'A task-centred group approach to work with the chronically mentally ill', *Social Work with Groups*, 15, 67–80.

Gelder, M., Gath, D. and Mayou, R. (1989) *Oxford Textbook of Psychiatry*, 2nd edn, Oxford: Oxford University Press.

George, L.K. and Gwyther, L.P. (1986) 'Caregiver well-being: A multidimensional examination of family caregivers of demented adults', *The Gerontologist*, 26, 253–9.

George, M. (1995) 'Vital recall', *Community Care*, 9–15 March, 16–17.

Getz, W., Wiesen, A.E., Sue, S. and Ayers, A. (1974) *Fundamentals of Crisis Counseling*, Lexington, MA: Lexington Books.

Gibbons, J., Bow, I., Butler, J. and Powell, J. (1979) 'Clients' reactions to task-centred casework: A follow-up study', *British Journal of Social Work*, 9, 203–16.

Gibson, F. (1994a) *Reminiscence and Recall: A Guide to Good Practice*, London: Age Concern England.

Gibson, F. (1994b) 'What can reminiscence contribute to people with dementia?', in Bornat, J. (ed.) *Reminiscence Reviewed: Perspectives, Evaluations, Achievements*, Buckingham: Open University Press.

Gibson, F. (1997) 'Owning the past in dementia care: Creative engagement with others in the present', in Marshall, M. (ed.) *State of the Art in Dementia Care*, London: Centre for Policy on Ageing.

Gilleard, C.J. (1984) *Living with Dementia*, London: Croom Helm.

Gilliard, J. (1997) 'Between a rock and a hard place: the impact of dementia on young carers', in Marshall, M. (ed.) *State of the Art in Dementia Care*, London: Centre for Policy on Ageing.

Gillies, C. and James, A. (1994) *Reminiscence Work with Old People*, London: Chapman and Hall.

Goffman, E. (1961) *Asylums: Essays on the Social Situation of Mental Patients and Other Inmates*, New York: Anchor Books.

Golan, N. (1978) *Treatment in Crisis Situations*, New York: Free Press.

Goldberg, D. and Huxley, P. (1992) *Common Mental Disorders. A Bio-social Approach*, London: Routledge.

Goldberg, E. and Connelly, N. (eds) (1981) *Evaluative Research in Social Care*, London: Heinemann Educational Books.

Goldberg, E.M., Walker, D. and Robinson, J. (1977) 'Exploring the task-centred casework method', *Social Work Today*, 9, 9–14.

Goldsmith, M. (1996) *Hearing the Voice of People with Dementia: Opportunities and Obstacles*, London: Jessica Kingsley.

Goldsmith, M. (1997) 'Hearing the voice of people with dementia', in Marshall, M. (ed.) *State of the Art in Dementia Care*, London: Centre for Policy on Ageing.

Grafstrom, M., Norberg, A. and Wimblad, B. (1992) 'Abuse is in the eye of the beholder: Reports by family members about abuse of demented persons in home care. A total population-based study', *Scandinavian Journal of Social Medicine*, 21, 247–55.

Gray, E. (1987) 'Brief task-centred casework in a crisis intervention team in a psychiatric setting', *Journal of Social Work Practice*, 3, 111–28.

Griffiths, R. (1988) *Community Care: Agenda for Action*, London: HMSO.

Gubrium, J.F. (1986) *Oldtimers and Alzheimer's: The Descriptive Organization of Senility*, London: JAI Press.

Gubrium, J.F. and Lynott, R.J. (1985) 'Alzheimer's disease as biographical work', in Peterson, W.A. and Quadagno, J. (eds) *Social Bonds in Later Life*, Beverly Hills, CA: Sage.

Guydish, J. and Kramer, J. (1982) 'Behaviour modification: Doing battle in the ethical arena', *Journal of Behaviour Therapy and Experimental Psychology*, 13, 315–20.

Gwyther, L.P., Lowenthal, R.I. and Marrazzo, R.A. (1990) 'Milestoning: Evoking memories for resocialization through group reminiscence', *Gerontologist*, 30, 269–72.

Hadley, R. and Hatch, S. (1981) *Social Welfare and the Failure of the State*, London: George Allen and Unwin.

Hall, G.S. (1922) *Senescence: The Last Half of Life*, London and New York: D. Appleton.

Hargrave, T.D. (1994) 'Using video life reviews with older adults', *Journal of Family Therapy*, 16, 259–68.

Harris, D.K. (1988) *Dictionary of Gerontology*, New York: Greenwood Press.

Hartmann, H. (1958) *Ego Psychology and the Problem of Adaptation*, New York: International University Press.

Harvey, M. (1990) *Who's Confused?*, Birmingham: PEPAR.

Hawton, K., Salkovskis, P.M., Kirk, J. and Clark, D.M. (eds) (1989) *Cognitive Behaviour Therapy for Psychiatric Problems: A Practical Guide*, Oxford: Oxford University Press.

Hawton, M., Hughes, G. and Percy-Smith, J. (1994) *Community Profiling*, Buckingham: Open University Press.

Hayek, F.A. (1960) *The Constitution of Liberty*, London: Routledge and Kegan Paul.

Hayes, G., Goodwin, T. and Miars, B. (1990) 'After disaster: A crisis support team at work', *American Journal of Nursing*, 90, 61–4.

Heap, K. (1977) *Group Theory for Social Workers: An introduction*, Oxford: Pergamon.

Henderson, A.S. (1986) 'The epidemiology of Alzheimer's disease', *British Medical Bulletin*, 42, 3–10.

Hodgkinson, P.E. and Stewart, M. (1991) *Coping with Catastrophe: A Handbook of Disaster Management*, London: Routledge

Hoff, L.A. (1989) *People in Crisis*, 3rd edn, Menlo Park, CA: Addison-Wesley.

Hoff, L.A. (1990) *Battered Women as Survivors*, London: Routledge.

Holden, U. and Woods, R. (1988) *Reality Orientation*, 2nd edn, New York: Churchill Livingstone.

Hollis, F. (1967) 'Principles and assumptions underlying casework practice', in Younghusband, E. (ed.) *Social Work and Social Values*, London: Allen and Unwin.

Homer, A. and Gilleard, C. (1990) 'Abuse of elderly people by their carers', *British Medical Journal*, 301, 1,359–62.

Howe, D. (1987) *An Introduction to Social Work Theory*, Aldershot: Wildwood House.

Hudson, B. and Macdonald, G. (1986) *Behavioural Social Work: An Introduction*, Basingstoke: Macmillan.

Hunter, S. (ed.) (1997) *Dementia: Challenges and New Directions*, London: Jessica Kingsley.

Hwalek, M, Sengstock, M. and Lawrence, R. (1986) 'Assessing the probability of abuse of the elderly', *Journal of Applied Gerontology*, 5, 153–73.

Jack, R. (1992) 'Institutionalised elder abuse, social work and social services departments', *Baseline*, 50, 24–7.

Jones, C. (1995a) 'Demanding social work education: An agenda for the end of the century', *Issues in Social Work Education*, 15, 3–17.

Jones, C. (1995b) '"Take me away from all this"… Can reminiscence be therapeutic in an intensive care unit?', *Intensive and Critical Care Nursing*, 11, 341–3.

Jones, G.M.M. and Miesen, B.M.L. (eds) (1992) *Caregiving in Dementia*, London: Routledge.

Jones, S. and Joss, R. 'Models of professionalism', in Yelloly, M. and Henkel, M. (eds) *Learning and Teaching in Social Work: Towards Reflective Practice*, London: Jessica Kingsley.

Jorm, A.F. (1987) *Understanding Senile Dementia*, London: Croom Helm.

Kaplan, S.G. and Wheeler, E.G. (1983) 'Survival skills for working with potentially violent clients', *Social Casework*, 64, 339–45.

Kay, D.W.K. (1991) 'The epidemiology of dementia: A review of recent work', *Reviews in Clinical Gerontology*, 1, 55–66.

Keady, J. (1997) 'Maintaining involvement: A meta concept to describe the dynamics of dementia', in Marshall, M. (ed.) *State of the Art in Dementia Care*, London: Centre for Policy on Ageing.

Kelly, G.A. (1955) *The Theory of Personal Constructs*, Vol. 1, New York: W.W. Norton.

King's Fund (1987) *Facilitating Innovation in Community Care*, London: King's Fund.

Kitwood, T. (1988) 'The technical, the personal and the framing of dementia', *Social Behaviour*, 3, 161–80.

Kitwood, T. (1990) 'The dialectics of dementia: With particular reference to Alzheimer's disease', *Ageing and Society*, 10, 177–96.

Kitwood, T. (1997a) 'Personhood, dementia and dementia care', in Hunter, S. (ed.) *Dementia: Challenge and New Directions*, London: Jessica Kingsley.

Kitwood, T. (1997b) *Dementia Reconsidered: The Person Comes First*, Buckingham: Open University Press.

Kitwood, T. and Benson, S. (eds) (1995) *The New Culture of Dementia Care*, London: Hawker.

Kitwood, T. and Bredin, K. (1992) 'Towards a theory of dementia care: Personhood and well-being', *Ageing and Society*, 12, 269–87.

Kurrle, S.E., Sadler, P.M. and Cameron, I.D. (1992) 'Patterns of elder abuse', *Medical Journal of Australia*, 157, 673–6.

Laing, R.D. (1965) *The Divided Self: An Existential Study in Sanity and Madness*, Harmondsworth: Penguin.

Langsley, D. (1968) *Families in Crisis*, New York: Grune and Stratton.

Lapernieve, M.G. (1993) 'Education-coup-de-fil: 10 ans de travail preventif avec les familles', *The Social Worker*, 61, 101–4.

Lau, E. and Kosberg, J. (1979) 'Abuse of the elderly by informal care providers', *Aging*, 299: 10–15.

Leat, D. (1986) 'Privatisation and voluntarisation', *Quarterly Journal of Social Affairs*, 2, 290–1.

Lefcourt, H.M. (1976) *Locus of Control: Current Trends in Theory and Research*, Hillside, NJ: Erlbaum/Wiley.

Levin, E., Sinclair, I. and Gorbach, P. (1989) *Families, Services and Confusion in Old Age*, Aldershot: Avebury.

Levy, R. and Post, F. (eds) (1982) *The Psychiatry of Later Life*, Oxford: Blackwell.

Lindemann, E. (1944) 'Symptomatology and management of acute grief', *American Journal of Psychiatry*, 101, 141–8.

Lishman, W.A. (1987) *Organic Psychiatry: The Psychological Consequences of Cerebral Disorder*, 2nd edn, Oxford: Blackwell.

Lodge, B. (1988) *Handbook of Mental Disorders in Old Age*, Buckingham: Open University Press.

Long, C. (1981) 'Geriatric abuse', *Issues in Mental Health Nursing*, 3, 123–35.

Macdonald, G. and Sheldon, B. (1992) 'Contemporary studies of the effectiveness of social work', *British Journal of Social Work*, 22, 615–43.

Magee, J.J. (1994) 'Using themes from mystical traditions to enhance self-acceptance in life review groups', *Journal of Religious Gerontology*, 9, 63–72.

Malde, S. (1988) 'Guided autobiography: A counseling tool for older adults', *Journal of Counseling and Development*, 66, 290–3.

Manthorpe, J. (1995) 'Elder abuse and dementia', *Journal of Dementia Care*, November/December, 27–9.

Marshall, M. (1983) *Social Work with Old People*, Basingstoke: Macmillan.

Marshall, M. (ed.) (1990) *Working with Dementia*, Birmingham: Venture Press.

Marshall, M. (1996) *I Can't Place this Place at All: Working with People with Dementia and Their Carers*, Birmingham: Venture Press.

Marshall, M. (ed.) (1997) *State of the Art in Dementia Care*, London: Centre for Policy on Ageing.

Martin, J.M. (1989) 'Expanding reminiscence therapy with elderly mentally infirm patients', *British Journal of Occupational Therapy*, 52, 435–6.

Mayer, J. and Timms, N. (1970) *The Client Speaks*, London: Routledge and Kegan Paul.

Mayo, M. (1994) 'Community work', in Hanvey, C. and Philpot, T. (eds) *Practising Social Work*, London: Routledge.

McCarthy, M. (1990) *The New Politics of Welfare*, London: Macmillan.

McDonnell, A., McEvoy, J. and Dearden, R.L. (1994) 'Coping with violent situations in the caring environment', in Wykes, T. (ed.) *Violence and Health Care Professionals*, London: Chapman and Hall.

McGee, R. (1974) *Crisis Intervention in the Community*, Baltimore, MD: University Park Press.

McGowan, T.G. (1994) 'Mentoring-reminiscence: A conceptual and empirical analysis', *International Journal of Aging and Human Development*, 39, 321–36.

McInnis-Dittrich, K. (1996) 'Adapting life-review therapy for elderly female survivors of childhood sexual abuse', *Families in Society*, 77, 166–73.

Meacher, M. (1972) *Taken for a Ride*, Harlow: Longman.

Meichenbaum, D. (1977) *Cognitive Behavior Modification: An Integrative Approach*, New York: Plenum.

Miller, K. (1963) 'The concept of crisis: Current status and mental health implications', *Human Organization*, 22, 195–201.

Ministry of Health (1962) *A Hospital Plan for England and Wales*, Cmnd 1604, London: HMSO.

Mullender, A. and Ward, D. (1991) *Self-directed Groupwork: Users Take Action for Empowerment*, London: Whiting and Birch.

Murgatroyd, S. (1985) *Counselling and Helping*, London: Methuen/British Psychological Society.

Murphy, C. and Moyes, M. (1997) 'Life story work', in Marshall, M. (ed.) *State of the Art in Dementia Care*, London: Centre for Policy on Ageing.

Murphy, E. (1986) *Dementia and Mental Illness in the Old*, Basingstoke: Macmillan.

Namazi, K.H. and Haynes, S.R. (1994) 'Sensory stimuli reminiscence for patients with Alzheimer's disease: Relevance and implications', *Clinical Gerontologist*, 14, 29–46.

Nelson-Jones R. (1983) *Practical Counselling Skills*, London: Holt, Rinehart and Winston.

Netton, A. (1993) *A Positive Environment?*, Aldershot: Ashgate.

Newhill, C.E. (1993) 'Short-term treatment of a severely suicidal Japanese American client with schizoaffective disorder', *Families in Society*, 74, 503–7.

Nicol, A.R., Smith, J., Kay, B., Hall, D., Barlow, J.J. and Williams, B. (1988) 'A focused casework approach to the treatment of child abuse: A controlled comparison', *Journal of Child Psychology and Psychiatry*, 29, 703–11.

Nolan, M. (1993) 'Carer–dependent relationships and the prevention of elder abuse', in Decalmer, P. and Glendenning, F. (eds) *The Mistreatment of Older People*, London: Sage.

Norman, A. (1982) *Mental Illness in Old Age: Meeting the Challenge*, London: Centre for Policy on Ageing.

Norris, A. (1986) *Reminiscence with Elderly People*, Bicester: Winslow Press.

Ogg, J. (1993) 'Researching elder abuse in Britain', *Journal of Elder Abuse and Neglect* , 5, 37–54.

O'Hagan, K. (1986) *Crisis Intervention in Social Services*, Basingstoke: Macmillan.

O'Hagan, K. (ed) (1996) *Competence in Social Work Practice: A Practical Guide for Professionals*, London: Jessica Kingsley.

Olsen, M.R. (ed.) (1984) *Social Work and Mental Health*, London: Tavistock.

O'Malley, J.A., O'Malley, H.C., Everitt, D.E. and Sarson, D. (1984) 'Categories of family mediated abuse and neglect of elderly persons', *Journal of the American Geriatrics Society*, 35: 363–9.

Orme, J. and Glastonbury, B. (1993) *Care Management*, Basingstoke: Macmillan.

Orton, J.D., Allen, M. and Cook, J. (1989) 'Reminiscence groups with confused nursing center residents: An experimental study', *Social Work in Health Care*, 14, 73–86.

Ott, R.L. (1993) 'Enhancing validation through milestoning with sensory reminiscence', *Journal of Gerontological Social Work*, 20, 147–59.

Parad, H. (ed.) (1965) *Crisis Intervention: Selected Readings*, New York: Family Service Association of America.

Parker, G. (1990) *With Due Care and Attention: A Review of Research on Informal Care*, London: Family Policy Studies Centre.

Parker, J. (1992) 'Crisis intervention: A framework for social work with people with dementia and their carers', *Elders*, 1, 43–57.

Parker, J. (1993) 'Dementia, social work and ethical principles', *Baseline*, 52, 33–41.

Parker, J. (1995) 'An anti-oppressive practice framework for the practice placement in social work', *The Journal of Staff Development and Practice*, 4, 35–46.

Parker, J. and Randall, P. (1997a) *Using Social and Psychological Theories*, Birmingham: Open Learning Foundation/British Association of Social Workers.

Parker, J. and Randall, P. (1997b) *Using Behavioural Theories*, Birmingham: Open Learning Foundation/British Association of Social Workers.

Parkes, C.M. (1971) 'Psycho-social transitions: A field for study', *Social Science and Medicine*, 5, 101–15.

Parry, G. (1990) *Coping with Crises*, London: BPS Books/Routledge.

Paveza, G.J., Cohen, D., Eisdorfer, C., Freels, S., Semla, T., Ashford, J.W., Gorelick, P., Hirshman, R., Luchins, D. and Levy, P. (1992) 'Severe family violence and Alzheimer's disease: Prevalence and risk factors', *Gerontologist*, 32, 493–7.

Pavlov, I.P. (1927) *Conditioned Reflexes*, London: Oxford University Press.

Payne, M. (1991) *Modern Social Work Theory: A Critical Introduction*, Basingstoke: Macmillan.

Penn, B. (1994) 'Using patient biography to promote holistic care', *Nursing Times*, 90, 35–6.

Penhale, B. (1992) 'Elder abuse: An overview', *Elders*, 1, 36–48.

Penhale, B. (1993) 'The abuse of elderly people: Considerations for practice', *British Journal of Social Work*, 23, 95–112.

Percy Report (1957) *Report of the Royal Commission on the Law Relating to Mental Illness and Mental Deficiency 1954–57*, Cmnd 169, London: HMSO.

Perlman, H.H. (1957) *Social Casework: A Problem-solving Process*, Chicago: University of Chicago Press.

Perlman, H.H. (1986) 'The problem-solving model', in Turner, F.J. (ed.) *Social Work Treatment: Interlocking Theoretical Approaches*, New York: Free Press.

Perls, F., Hefferline, R.F. and Goodman, P. (1973) *Gestalt Therapy: Excitement and Growth in the Human Personality*, Harmondsworth: Penguin.

Phair, L. (1997) 'Elder abuse and dementia: Moving forward', in Marshall, M. (ed.) *State of the Art in Dementia Care*, London: Centre for Policy on Ageing.

Phillipson, C. and Biggs, S. (1995) 'Elder abuse: A critical overview', in Kingston, P.A. and Penhale, B. (eds) *Family Violence and the Caring Professions*, Basingstoke: Macmillan.

Pillemer, K.A. (1986) 'Risk factors in elder abuse: Results from a case-control study', in Pillemer, K.A. and Wolf, R.S. (eds) *Elder Abuse: Conflict in the Family*, Dover, MA: Auburn House.

Pillemer, K.A. and Suitor, J.J. (1988) 'Elder abuse', in Van Hasselt, V., Morrison, R., Belack A. and Hensen, M. (eds) *Handbook of Family Violence*, New York: Plenum Press.

Pillemer, K.A. and Suitor, J.J. (1992) 'Violence and violent feelings: What causes them among family caregivers?', *Journal of Gerontology*, 47, S165–S172.

Pillemer, K.A. and Wolf, R.S. (eds) (1986) *Elder Abuse: Conflict in the Family*, Dover, MA: Auburn House.

Podnieks, E. (1990) *National Survey on Abuse of the Elderly in Canada: The Ryerson Study*, Toronto: Ryerson Polytechnical Institute.

Pot, A.M., Van Dyck, R., Jonker, C. and Deeg, D.J.H. (1996) 'Verbal and physical aggression against demented elderly by informal caregivers in the Netherlands', *Journal of Social Psychiatry and Social Epidemiology*, 31, 156–62.

Quinn, M. and Tomita, S. (1986) *Elder Abuse and Neglect: Causes, Diagnosis and Intervention Strategies*, New York: Springer.

Raaijmakers, J. and Abbenhuis, M. (1992) 'Learning and memory in demented patients', in Jones, G.M.M. and Miesen, B.M.L. (eds) *Care-giving in Dementia: Research and Applications*, London and New York: Tavistock/Routledge.

Rabinowitz, J. and Lukoff, I. (1995) 'Clinical decision making of short- versus long-term treatment', *Research on Social Work Practice*, 5, 62–79.

Ramakrishnan, K.R. and Balgopal, P.R. (1992) 'Linking task-centred intervention with employee assistance programs', *Families in Society*, 73, 488–94.

Rapoport, L. (1970) 'Crisis intervention as a mode of brief treatment', in Roberts, R.W. and Nee, R.H. (eds) *Theories of Social Casework*, Chicago: University of Chicago Press.

Rathbone-McCuan, E., Travis, A. and Voyles, B. (1983) 'Family intervention: The task-centred approach,' in Kosberg, J.I. (ed.) *Abuse and Maltreatment of the Elderly: Causes and Interventions*, Boston, MA: J. Wright.

Rattenbury, C. and Stones, M.J. (1989) 'A controlled evaluation of reminiscence and current topics discussion groups in a nursing home context', *Gerontologist*, 29, 768–71.

Reay, A. (1997) 'The Use of Anger Management and Education as Intervention within Elder Abuse and Neglect' personal communication.

Reid, W. (1978) *The Task-centred System*, New York: Columbia University Press.

Reid, W. (1987) 'Evaluating an intervention in developmental research', *Journal of Social Service Research*, 11, 17–37.

Reid, W. and Epstein, L. (1972) *Task-centred Casework*, New York: Columbia University Press.

Reid, W. and Epstein, L. (eds) (1977) *Task-centred Practice*, New York: Columbia University Press.

Reid, W. and Helmer, K. (1985) *Session Tasks in Family Treatment*, New York: State University of New York at Albany.

Reid, W. and Shyne, A. (1969) *Brief and Extended Casework*, New York: Columbia University Press.

Reid, W. and Strother, P. (1988) 'Super problem solvers: A systematic case study', *Social Service Review*, 62, 430–45.

Riley P. (1993) cited in Social Services Inspectorate (1993) *No Longer Afraid: The Safeguard of Older People in Domestic Settings*, London: HMSO.

Riordan, J. and Whitmore, B. (1990) *Living with Dementia*, Manchester: Manchester University Press.

Roberts, A.R. (ed.) (1991) *Contemporary Perspectives on Crisis Intervention and Prevention*, Englewood Cliffs, NJ: Prentice-Hall.

Rogers, C. (1951) *Client-centred Therapy: Its Current Practice, Implications and Theory*, Boston, MA: Houghton-Mifflin.

Rogers, C. (1961) *On Becoming a Person*, Boston, MA: Houghton-Mifflin.

Rojek, C. and Collins, S. (1987) 'Contract or con trick?', *British Journal of Social Work*, 17, 199–211.

Rotter, J.B., Chance, J.E. and Phares, C.J. (1972) *Applications of a Social Learning Theory of Personality*, New York: Holt, Rienhart and Winston.

Royal College of Physicians (1981) 'Organic memory impairment in the elderly: Implications for research, education and the provision of services', *Journal of the Royal College of Physicians*, 15, 141–67.

Rybarczyk, B.D. and Auerbach, S.M. (1990) 'Reminiscence interviews as stress management interventions for older patients undergoing surgery', *Gerontologist*, 30, 522–8.

Sadler, P., Kurrle, S. and Cameron, I. (1995) 'Dementia and elder abuse', *Australian Journal on Ageing*, 14, 36–40.

Saleeby, D. (1996) 'The strengths perspective in social work practice: Extensions and cautions', *Social Work*, 41, 296–305.

Salisbury, B. (1989) 'Towards dignity and self-determination', *Service Brokerage*, 1, v–vi.

Saveman, B.I. and Norberg, A. (1993) 'Cases of elder abuse, intervention and hopes for the future, as reported by home service personnel', *Scandinavian Journal of Caring Science*, 7, 21–8.

Scheff, T.J. (1966) *On Being Mentally Ill*, London: Weidenfeld and Nicolson.

Schulz, R., O'Brien, A.T., Bookwala, J. and Fleissner, K. (1995) 'Psychiatric and physical morbidity effects of dementia caregiving: Prevalence, correlates and causes', *Gerontologist*, 35, 771–91.

Scott, E.K. (1993) 'How to stop the rapist? A question of strategy in two rape crisis centers', *Social Policy*, 40, 343–61.

Scrutton, R. (1989) *Counselling Older People*, London: Edward Arnold.

Seaton, M. (1994) 'A duty to care, control and restraint', *Elders*, 3, 5–13.

Seligman, M.E.P. (1975) *Helplessness*, San Francisco, CA: Freeman.

Sheldon, B. (1982) *Behaviour Modification: Theory, Practice and Philosophy*, London: Tavistock.

Sheldon, B. (1986) 'Social work effectiveness experiments: Review and implications', *British Journal of Social Work*, 16, 223–42.

Sheldon, B. (1995) *Cognitive-behavioural Therapy: Research, Practice and Philosophy*, London: Routledge.

Sherman, E. and Peak, T. (1991) 'Patterns of reminiscence and the assessment of late life adjustment', *Journal of Gerontological Social Work*, 16, 59–74.

Sinason, V. (1992) *Mental Handicap and the Human Condition: New Approaches from the Tavistock*, London: Free Association Books.

Snell, J. (1991) 'Reviving memories', *Nursing Times*, 87, 54–6.

Solomon, B.B. (1976) *Black Empowerment: Social Work in Oppressed Communities*, New York: Columbia University Press.

SSI (Social Services Inspectorate) (1991) *Care Management and Assessment*, London: HMSO.

SSI (Social Services Inspectorate) (1992) *Confronting Elder Abuse*, London: HMSO.

Stearns, P. (1986) 'Old age family conflict: The perspective of the past', in Pillemer, K.A. and Wolf, R.S. (eds) *Elder Abuse: Conflict in the Family*, Dover, MA: Auburn House.

Steinmetz, S.K. (1990) 'Elder abuse: Myth and reality', in Brubaker, T.H. (ed.) *Family Relationships in Later Life*, 2nd edn, Newbury Park, CA: Sage.

Stevenson, D.G. and Grauerholz, E. (1993) 'The role of crisis centers in defining and reporting child abuse', *Families in Society*, 74, 195–203.

Stokes, G. (1987a) *Aggression*, Bicester: Winslow Press.

Stokes, G. (1987b) *Incontinence and Inappropriate Urinating*, Bicester: Winslow Press.

Stokes, G. (1987c) *Screaming and Shouting*, Bicester: Winslow Press.

Stokes, G. (1987d) *Wandering*, Bicester: Winslow Press.

Suitor, J.J. and Pillemer, K.A. (1993) 'Support and interpersonal stress in the social networks of married daughters caring for parents with dementia', *Journal of Gerontology*, 48, S1–S8.

Sutton, C. (1994) *Social Work, Community Work and Psychology*, Leicester: BPS Books.

Sutton L.J. and Cheston, R. (1997) 'Rewriting the story of dementia: A narrative approach to psychotherapy with people with dementia', in Marshall, M. (ed.) *State of the Art in Dementia Care*, London: Centre for Policy on Ageing.

Szasz, T.S. (1971) *The Manufacture of Madness*, London: Routledge and Kegan Paul.

Szasz, T.S. (1974) *The Myth of Mental Illness*, New York: Harper and Row.

Tabourne, C.E.S. (1995a) 'The effects of a life review program on disorientation, social interaction and self-esteem of nursing home residents', *International Journal of Aging and Human Development*, 41, 251–66.

Tabourne, C.E.S. (1995b) 'The life review program as an intervention for an older adult newly admitted to a nursing home facility: A case study', *Therapeutic Recreation Journal*, 29, 228–36.

Taft, L.B. and Nehrke, M.F. (1990) 'Reminiscence, life review, and ego integrity in nursing home residents', *International Journal of Aging and Human Development*, 30, 189–96.

Tamayo, L., January, G., Peet, M. and Benditssky, H. (1990) 'The systems impact of an urban mobile crisis team', in Cohen, N.L. (ed.) *Psychiatry Takes to the Streets: Outreach and Crisis Intervention for the Mentally Ill*, New York and London: Guilford Press.

Thompson, N. (1993) *Anti-discriminatory Practice*, Basingstoke: Macmillan.

Thompson, N. (1991) *Crisis Intervention Revisited*, Birmingham: PEPAR.

Timms, N. (1983) *Social Work Values: An Enquiry*, London: Routledge and Kegan Paul.

Toft, B. and Reynolds, S. (1994) *Learning from Disasters*, Oxford: Butterworth/Heinemann.

Tuckman, B.W. (1965) 'Developmental sequences in small groups', *Psychological Bulletin*, 63, 384–99.

Turner, B. (1987) *Medical Power and Social Knowledge*, London: Sage.

Twelvetrees, A. (1991) *Community Work*, London: Macmillan.

Twigg, J., Atkin, K. and Perring, C. (1990) *Carers and Services: A Review of Research*, London: HMSO.

Vass, A.A. (ed.) (1996) *Social Work Competences: Core Knowledge, Values and Skills*, London: Sage.

Wagner Report (1988) *Residential Care: A Positive Choice*, London: HMSO.

Watson, J.B. and Raynor, R. (1920) 'Conditioned emotional reactions', *Journal of Experimental Psychology*, 3, 1–14.

Webb, N.B. (ed.) (1991) *Play Therapy with Children in Crisis*, New York and London: Guilford Press.

Webster, J.D. (1993) 'Construction and validation of the reminiscence functions scale', *Journal of Gerontology*, 48, 256–62.

Webster, J.D. and Young, R.A. (1988) 'Process variables of the life review: Counseling implications', *International Journal of Aging and Human Development*, 26, 315–23.

Whitaker, D.S. (1985) *Using Groups to Help People*, London: Routledge and Kegan Paul.

Wilcock, G. (1990) *Living with Alzheimer's Disease*, London: Penguin.

Wilson, G. (1994) 'Abuse of elderly men and women among clients of a community psychogeriatric service', *British Journal of Social Work*, 24, 681–700.

Winner, M. (1992) *Quality Work with Older People*, London: Central Council for Education and Training in Social Work.

Wolf, R.S. (1986) 'Major findings from three model projects on elder abuse', in Pillemer, K.A. and Wolf, R.S. (eds) (1986) *Elder Abuse: Conflict in the Family*, Dover, MA: Auburn House.

Wolf, R. and Pillemer, K. (1989) *Helping Elderly Victims*, New York: Columbia University Press.

Woods, R. (1995) 'The beginnings of a new culture in care', in Kitwood, T. and Benson, S. (eds) *The New Culture of Dementia Care*, London: Hawker.

Woolley, N. (1990) 'Crisis theory: A paradigm of effective intervention with families of critically ill people', *Journal of Advanced Nursing*, 15, 1402–8.

Wynne-Harley, D. (1991) *Living Dangerously: Risk-taking and Older People*, London: Centre for Policy on Ageing.

Yale, R. (1996) *Developing Support Groups for Individuals with Early-stage Alzheimer's Disease: Planning, Implementation and Evaluation*, London: Jessica Kingsley.

Yelloly, M. (1995) 'Professional competence and higher education', in Yelloly, M. and Hankel, M. (eds) *Learning and Teaching in Social Work*, London: Jessica Kingsley.

Index